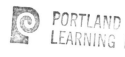

Color Atlas of

THE EYE IN CLINICAL MEDICINE

Joseph B. Michelson
MD FACS
Director, Retina–Uveitis Service
Head, Division of Ophthalmology
Scripps Clinic and Research Foundation
La Jolla, California, USA

Consultant in Retina and Uveitis
US Naval Regional Medical Center
San Diego, USA

Mitchell H. Friedlaender
MD
Director, Cornea and Refractive Surgery
Scripps Clinic and Research Foundation
La Jolla, California, USA

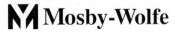 Mosby-Wolfe

London Baltimore Barcelona Bogotá Boston Buenos Aires Caracas Carlsbad, CA Chicago Madrid Mexico City Milan Naples, FL New York
Philadelphia St. Louis Seoul Singapore Sydney Taipei Tokyo Toronto Wiesbaden

Copyright © 1996 Times Mirror International Publishers Limited

Published in 1996 by Mosby-Wolfe, an imprint of Times Mirror International Publishers Limited

Printed by Grafos S.A. arte sobre papel, Barcelona, Spain.

ISBN 0 7234 2147 1

For full details of all Times Mirror International Publishers Limited titles, please write to Times Mirror International Publishers Limited, Lynton House, 7–12 Tavistock Square, London WC1H 9LB, England.

A CIP catalogue record for this book is available from the British Library.

Library of Congress Cataloging-in-Publication Data Applied For

Project Manager:	Paul Phillips
Developmental Editor:	Lucy Hamilton
Layout:	Lindy van den Berghe
Cover Design:	Ian Spick
Illustration:	Paul Bernson
Production:	Siobhan Egan
Index:	John Gibson
Publisher:	Geoff Greenwood

Contents

Preface

The study of medicine in general and ophthalmology in particular has been truly advanced over the immediate past 25 years through the enhanced visualization of the fundus of the eye. Indirect ophthalmoscopy, slit-lamp biomicroscopy, especially with different high power lenses, flourescein angiography, indocyanine green angiography, the imaging techniques of CAT scan and MRI have all brought the eye and its circulation under intense scholastic scrutiny. And the yield to clinicians and researchers has been nothing short of bountiful. We have all been introduced into an ever-expanding world of histopathology up close and observable. We directly visualize the vasculitis of collagen-vascular disease, the infarction of the retinal and nerve tissue in AIDs and hypertensive disease, the microangiopathy of diabetes as it affects the body in general and a multitude of infections that invade the body but are under direct observation in the eye.

The eye is a unique point of departure in the investigation of systemic disease, and as ophthalmologists it is especially incumbent upon us to serve as your travel guide. We hope that both ophthalmologists, ophthalmologists-in-training, and our non-ophthalmic medical associates enjoy the trip in this volume!

JBM and MHF
February 1995

I would like to dedicate this volume to G. Richard O'Connor MD and Robert A Nozik MD who helped to shape my personal knowledge of ophthamology and my love of humanity.

J.B.M.

1.
Connective Tissue Diseases

The arthritides and the collagen vascular diseases share many ocular manifestations:
- dry eyes;
- iridocyclitis;
- episcleritis;
- an underlying histological feature of vasculitis.

RHEUMATOID ARTHRITIS

While rheumatoid arthritis is not usually an arthritis-associated uveitis syndrome (like ankylosing spondylitis, Reiter's syndrome, and juvenile rheumatoid arthritis), it can be a cause of contiguous iridocyclitis when it occurs in association with a scleritis, episcleritis, or an inflamed scleral nodule involving the limbus (**1.1–1.7, Table 1.1**).

Some of the very severe melting syndromes such as keratomalacia may occur near the limbus and can stimulate a secondary iridocyclitis. Dry eye syndrome or keratitis sicca is the most common eye manifestation associated with rheumatoid arthritis.

Rheumatoid arthritis is a chronic progressive polyarthritis that occurs three times more commonly in women. The average age of onset is between 30 and 40 years. There is a familial tendency and joint deformities are the rule. Keratitis sicca, scleritis, and sclerokeratitis are the main ophthalmic manifestations, but a troublesome, nongranulomatous iritis may occur with these conditions in rare cases.

Extra-articular manifestations of rheumatoid arthritis include pericarditis, pleuritis, nodular pulmonary disease, interstitial fibrosis of the lungs, muscle atrophy,

Rheumatoid arthritis
Definition • Secondary iridocyclitis (usually episcleritis) • Primary corneal melt (ischaemia)
Presentation • Iridocyclitis • Nongranulomatous
Investigation • Positive rheumatoid factor latex fixation test • Erythrocyte sedimentation rate • Joint radiograph
Therapy • Local intensive corticosteroids • Periocular • Short course high-dose systemic corticosteroids • Antimetabolites • Cyclosporin
Prognosis • Sometimes good • Sometimes poor

Table 1.1 Rheumatoid arthritis.

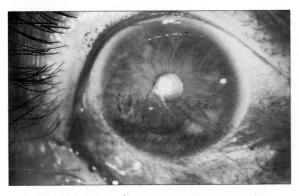

1.1 Typical dry eye syndrome is demonstrated by rose bengal staining of the cornified epithelium of the conjunctiva and the corneal limbus.

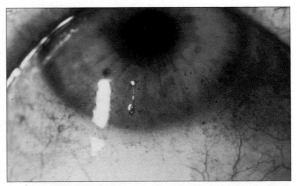

1.2 Filamentary keratitis may be prominent secondary to keratitis sicca, as seen here with a filament on the inferior cornea highlighted by rose bengal staining in the conjunctiva in and around the limbus.

lymphadenopathy, splenomegaly, and rheumatoid nodules. Interestingly, the vasculitis, which is seen with peripheral neuropathy, is not a feature in the retina. The cutaneous manifestations include purpura, splinter haemorrhages, skin infection due to vascular necrosis, ulceration, and digital gangrene.

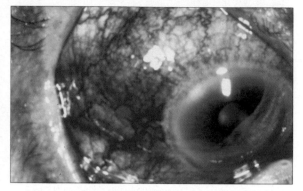

1.3 Nodular scleritis occurring near the limbus. This is a cause of secondary iritis.

1.4 Episcleritis and scleritis. An intensely injected conjunctiva and episclera is the rule with a diffuse rheumatoid scleral uveitis.

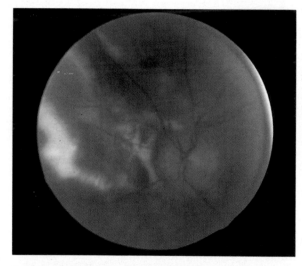

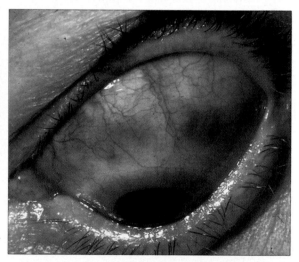

1.5 Uveal effusion. Fundus of patient with uveal effusion due to posterior nodular scleritis caused by rheumatoid disease. This is frequently confused with malignant melanoma of the choroid.

1.6 A mild scleral ectasia associated with advanced crippling rheumatoid arthritis.

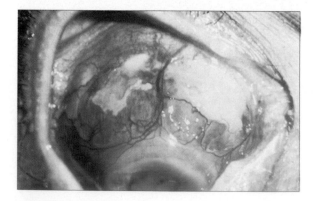

1.7 Profound keratomalacia perforans with almost no residual sclera compounded by a profound uveitis with a cloudy cornea. The scleral/corneal melting is not amenable to surgical repair because there is no anterior tissue into which a possible scleral graft can be sewn. (Courtesy of Will's Eye Hospital, Residents Teaching Collection.)

JUVENILE RHEUMATOID ARTHRITIS

Juvenile rheumatoid arthritis (**Table 1.2**) is not a childhood variety of adult rheumatoid arthritis. It is a different disease and may be a chronic and progressive crippler of children. Onset is usually from 2 to 4 years of age. More common in young girls than boys, it rarely manifests itself before the age of 6 months. Iridocyclitis and the associated ocular complications of cataract and glaucoma are frequent causes of blindness in these children and may overshadow the acute initial episode of arthritis over a long period. Since cataract or iridocyclitis can occur in a quiet, white eye much as with pars planitis, accurate identification of this syndrome is essential (**1.8–1.15**).

There are three distinct types of juvenile rheumatoid arthritis:
- Still's disease;
- polyarticular juvenile rheumatoid arthritis;
- monoarticular or pauciarticular juvenile rheumatoid arthritis.

Paradoxically, ocular inflammation is rare when the systemic disease is most severe and it is the monoarticular or pauciarticular variety of juvenile rheumatoid arthritis that has the most severe forms of ocular complications. Frequently the systemic illness may be so mild as to escape detection, but ocular complications may occur in up to 25% of patients with the monoarticular or pauciarticular variety of juvenile rheumatoid arthritis.

Juvenile rheumatoid arthritis

Definition
- Chronic iridocyclitis

Presentation
- Iridocyclitis
- Nongranulomatous

Investigation
- Antinuclear antibody
- Erythrocyte sedimentation rate
- Paediatric rheumatological consultation

Therapy
- Medium-strength mydriatic/cycloplegic agent, at least nightly, even in remission
- More frequent mydriatic/cycloplegics during exacerbations
- Periocular corticosteroids
- Systemic corticosteroids during exacerbations
- Some patients do well on low-dose chronic systemic corticosteroids
- Cyclosporin contraindicated
- Antimetabolites are usually contraindicated

Complications
- Cataracts
- Band keratopathy
- Phthisis bulbi

Prognosis
- Variable

Table 1.2 Juvenile rheumatoid arthritis.

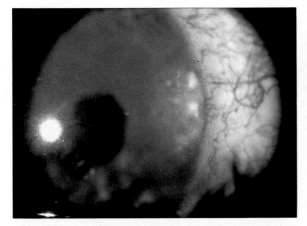

1.8 Recurrent flare-up of intense iridocyclitis with large white keratic precipitates. This 24-year-old woman has constant typical low-grade iritis secondary to juvenile rheumatoid arthritis. Note the 'early' band keratopathy changes temporally.

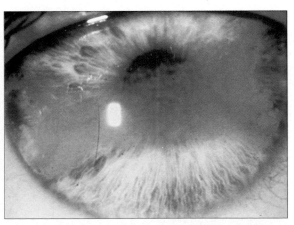

1.9 Band keratopathy. This was ongoing indolent clinically unrecognized iridocyclitis in an otherwise white, typically quiet eye of a child with juvenile rheumatoid arthritis.

Still's disease is the classical febrile severe illness with large joint involvement, lymphadenopathy, and splenomegaly and may be confused with mononucleosis. It may only occasionally cause iridocyclitis with apparent ocular manifestations. The polyarticular type of juvenile rheumatoid arthritis accounts for 50% of the children with this disease. Still's disease is usually seen in young children, but few have iridocyclitis or other ocular involvement.

Patients with mild or no history of monoarticular or pauciarticular arthritis, but who have signs of iridocyclitis with synechiae, secondary glaucoma, and cataracts, and more importantly, band keratopathy as a presenting sign, should be considered to have juvenile rheumatoid arthritis until proven otherwise. The iridocyclitis is essentially nongranulomatous, but small and fine keratic precipitates are usually present. It is typically indolent and the eye is usually neither injected nor painful. For these reasons, iridocyclitis may go unnoticed by family physicians and parents until the vision is so reduced that it is only discovered by a routine eye examination.

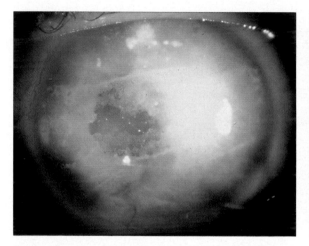

1.10 Intense iridocyclitis with profound overlying band keratopathy changes in the cornea of a 22-year-old woman whose other eye suffered from phthisis bulbi, indicating the profound ocular disease that can be manifested in these otherwise young, seemingly healthy patients with juvenile rheumatoid arthritis.

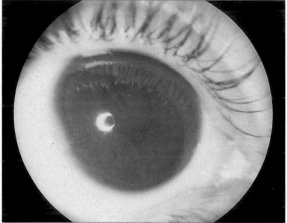

1.11 Cyclitic membrane formed after cataract surgery in a child with juvenile rheumatoid arthritis. These eyes used to be considered poor candidates for cataract surgery; however, with the advent of pars plana vitrectomy techniques these eyes can be successfully operated on for cataract and cyclitic membrane. Many avoid the development of phthisis bulbi, which is a consequence of ciliary body detachment from the 360° circular pulling of a cyclitic membrane on the ciliary body eventually resulting in hypotony and eventual phthisis.

1.12 Monoarticular arthritis in the hand of a small child with juvenile rheumatoid arthritis and concomitant iridocyclitis, cataract, and synechiae.

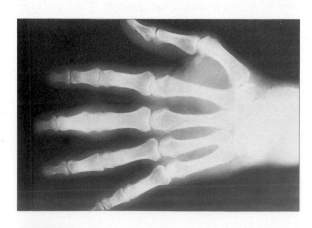

Posterior segment inflammation is very unusual, but choroiditis has been noted and vitreous floaters may be common.

When a child presents with such a quiet white eye with band keratopathy, synechiae, and vitreous cells, *Toxocara canis* must also be ruled out. Pars planitis usually presents in older children, and synechiae and

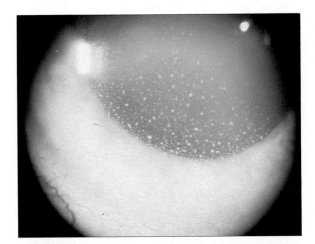

1.13 **Small fine white keratic precipitates** in a child with early cataract formation and iridocyclitis with a juvenile rheumatoid arthritis picture.

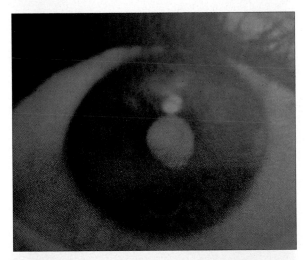

1.14 **Dense white cataract and synechiae** in a patient with monoarticular juvenile rheumatoid arthritis.

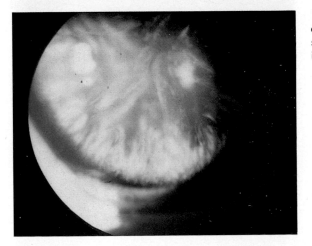

1.15 **Dense anterior subcapsular nuclear-sclerotic and posterior subcapsular cataract** in a patient whose synechiae were broken with dilation from an early and acute iridocyclitis with juvenile rheumatoid arthritis.

 PORTLAND COMMUNITY COLLEGE
LEARNING RESOURCE CENTERS

band keratopathy are frequently absent. Children with juvenile rheumatoid arthritis are usually seronegative for rheumatoid factor and positive for antinuclear antibody.

ANKYLOSING SPONDYLITIS

Ankylosing spondylitis (**1.16–1.18, Table 1.3**) is most common in men in their 20s and 30s. The eye disease may be unilateral, but often occurs in both eyes,

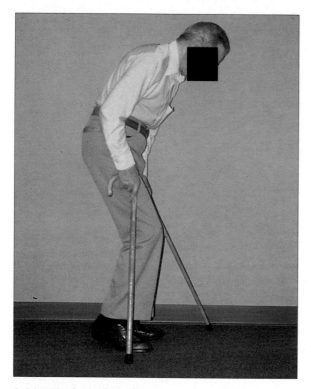

1.16 Marie-Strümpell spine. A man with ankylosing spondylitis demonstrating the typical stooped posture of the Marie-Strümpell spine.

Ankylosing spondylitis
Definition • Acute intermittent iridocyclitis
Presentation • Iridocyclitis • Nongranulomatous
Investigation • HLA B27 (positive > 90%) • Erythrocyte sedimentation rate • Sacroiliac joint radiographs
Therapy • Intensive local corticosteroids • Pupillary dilatation • Periocular corticosteroids, if severe • No treatment between attacks
Complications • Cataracts • Posterior synechiae • Glaucoma • Rarely, phthisis bulbi
Prognosis • Good • Poor, if chronic

Table 1.3 Ankylosing spondylitis.

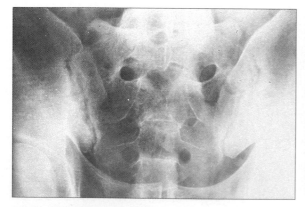

1.17 Sacroiliac sclerosis. Sacroiliac radiographs show sclerosis and blurring of the margins of the sacroiliac joint in a patient with ankylosing spondylitis. In early spondylitis a ^{99m} technetium bone scan may be more sensitive in the absence of typical radiographic changes.

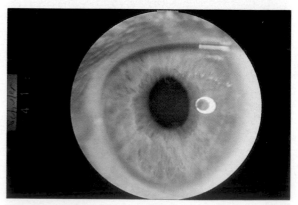

1.18 Notable Koeppe nodules on the iris margin from intermittent inflammation in an adolescent with ankylosing spondylitis.

though almost never concurrently. Iridocyclitis may precede clinical joint disease. In most patients, acute intermittent recurrent iridocyclitis is the rule. About half of all patients whose radiographs show evidence of ankylosing spondylitis are asymptomatic, so it is worth obtaining sacroiliac radiographs of all men with recurrent iridocyclitis, regardless of systemic complaints.

The HLA B27 antigen is positive in over 90% of patients, while the sedimentation rate is often elevated during an acute attack of spondylitis and tests for rheumatoid factor are negative.

REITER'S DISEASE

Reiter's disease consists of nonspecific urethritis with polyarthritis and conjunctivitis followed by recurrent iridocyclitis (**1.19–1.22, Table 1.4**) and is most common in men. Cutaneous mucosal lesions may cause confusion with Behçet's disease. Most patients are 20–40 years of age.

The first ocular sign may be papillary conjunctivitis, which occurs in up to one-third of cases. The ocular signs that follow are most often iritis and recurrent iridocyclitis. There may be severe pain, photophobia, diminished vision, synechiae, keratic precipitates, and large numbers of cells in the

Reiter's disease

Definition
- Acute intermittent iridocyclitis

Presentation
- Iridocyclitis
- Nongranulomatous

Investigation
- HLA B27 (positive 80%)
- Erythrocyte sedimentation rate
- Radiographs
- Rheumatological consultation

Therapy
- Intensive local corticosteroids
- Pupillary dilatation

Complications
- Cataracts
- Posterior synechiae
- Glaucoma
- Rarely, phthisis, if chronic

Prognosis
- Excellent (often begins with papillary conjunctivitis)

Table 1.4 Reiter's disease.

1.19 Large papillary conjunctivitis in a 12-year-old patient with Reiter's disease.

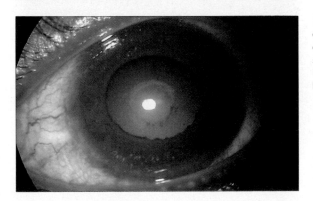

1.20 Vossius' ring. Eye of young African–American adolescent with concomitant sickle cell disease and Reiter's disease, demonstrating Vossius' ring from which he had synechiae for 360° on the anterior lens capsule. Note the irregularly formed pupillary margin with multiple areas of Koeppe nodulation and broken synechiae.

anterior chamber and the anterior vitreous. Keratitis and episcleritis may also occur.

The systemic signs of Reiter's syndrome are non-specific culture-negative urethritis and cystitis, which can lead to chronic prostatitis and recurrent urinary tract inflammations. The arthropathic manifestations are usually inflammation of the large weight-bearing joints, particularly the ankles and knees, and there seems to be some later overlap with an arthritic picture similar to ankylosing spondylitis. A cutaneous inflammation of keratoderma blennorrhagica occurs in less than 10% of patients, while mucosal lesions affecting the mouth and genitalia occur in 25%.

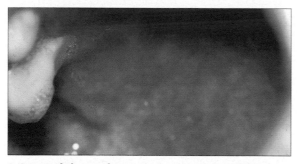

1.21 Aphthous ulcer in the buccal mucosa of a patient with Reiter's disease demonstrating the confusion that may arise between this diagnostic entity and Behçet's disease.

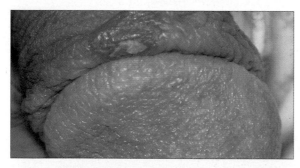

1.22 Aphthous ulceration on the penile shaft in this 24-year-old white male with Reiter's disease, confusing this entity with Behçet's disease.

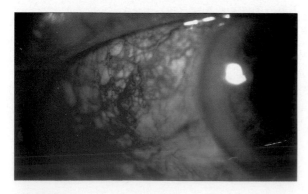

RELAPSING POLYCHONDRITIS

Relapsing polychondritis (chronic atrophic polychondritis, **1.23–1.30, Table 1.5**) is an uncommon arthritic disorder characterized by recurrent inflammation in cartilaginous tissues throughout the body. It occurs in both sexes and usually has its onset at between 20 and 60 years of age. Its pathogenesis is unknown, but it is often classified with the other collagen vascular and connective tissue diseases.

Inflammation of the pinnae of the ears is the most common feature of this disorder, and one or both become red, swollen, and painful. Repeated attacks

Relapsing polychondritis

Definition
• Papillary conjunctivitis
• Iridocyclitis

Presentation
• Initial papillary conjunctivitis followed by iridocyclitis
• Iridocyclitis, keratitis, keratouveitis
• Episcleritis, scleritis
• Nongranulomatous

Investigation
• Physical examination (cartilage absent, floppy ears, decreased nasal cartilage)

Therapy
• Topical corticosteroids
• Immunosuppressives (especially chlorambucil)
• Cyclosporin

Complications
• Corneal scarring

Prognosis
• Good

Table 1.5 Relapsing polychondritis.

1.23 Diffuse scleritis in a patient with relapsing polychondritis.

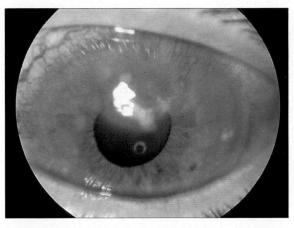

1.24   Thickened corneal epithelial disruption and scarring with acute episcleritis and scleritis in a patient with relapsing polychondritis.

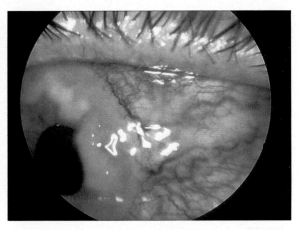

1.25   Diffuse corneal changes with acute epithelial dehiscence and adjacent necrotizing scleritis in a 24-year-old professional ballerina with relapsing polychondritis.

1.26   Other eye of ballerina in 1.25 with corneal epithelial changes, iritis and very deep, intensely painful episcleritis and scleritis.

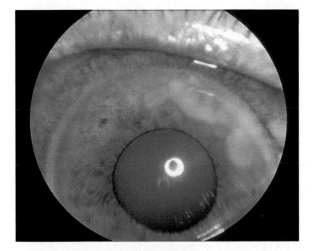

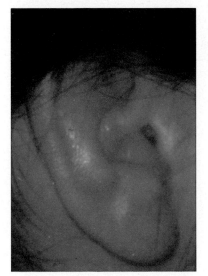

1.27   Acutely painful, hot erythematous, swollen pinna of patient in **1.25** with acute relapsing polychondritis.

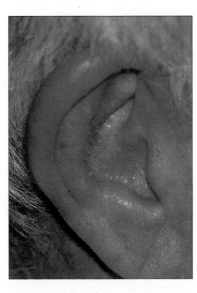

1.28   Cartilaginous resorption of 'floppy' pinna of a middle-aged male who had had many bouts of acute relapsing polychondritis.

lead to resorption of ear cartilage and floppy, drooping ears.

Arthralgias and arthritis are common. Inflammation and resorption of the nasal cartilage is also a frequent finding, sometimes resulting in a saddle-nose deformity. A number of systemic diseases have been found in association with this disorder, including vasculitis, rheumatoid arthritis, systemic and discoid lupus erythematosus, ankylosing spondylitis, ulcerative colitis, and sarcoidosis.

There may be considerable overlap between the types of uveitis aetiology in patients who present with these unusual connective tissue manifestations. Episcleritis is probably the commonest complication, but conjunctivitis and keratitis occur as well. Scleritis may involve primarily the anterior portions of the eye and many patients often have an associated keratoconjunctivitis sicca. Involvement of the retina and optic nerve is seen far less often than the anterior ocular complications. However, there are several

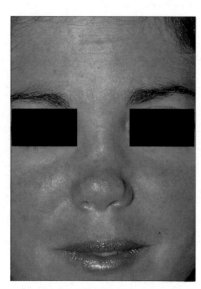

1.29 Note the resorbed nasal cartilage of a 24-year-old female with relapsing polychondritis.

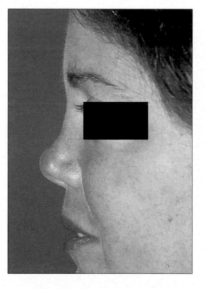

1.30 Profile of patient in 1.29 showing 'ski jump' side view of her nose resulting from resorbed nasal cartilage.

reports of associated active and inactive chorio-retinopathy, and there is one case in which the clinical picture is similar to that of a juvenile Coats' disease. Optic neuritis has also been reported.

COLLAGEN VASCULAR DISEASES (CONNECTIVE TISSUE INFLAMMATION)

The collagen vasculoses (**Table 1.6**) include lupus erythematosus, polyarteritis nodosum, Wegener's disease, and chronic relapsing polychondritis, and are systemic inflammatory disorders that may produce a vasculitis in the posterior pole of the eye. This retinal and/or choroidal vasculitis may simulate conditions such as Behçet's disease, Vogt–Koyanagi–Harada disease, syphilis, and tuberculosis.

The ocular findings include butterfly eruptions and purpuras on the lids and maxilla as well as telangiectases and true vasculitis. Keratitis sicca may be present in about one-third of the patients.

Corneal punctate epithelial keratitis as well as deep disciform keratitis may be presenting signs and causes of photophobia, lacrimation, and ocular discomfort. Nodular necrotizing scleritis or corneal melt may be a prominent part of this disease, as it is especially in rheumatoid arthritis. Cotton wool spots called cytoid bodies may appear in the retina in up to 20% of patients. These are the consequences of occlusive vasculitis of the nerve fibre cell layer in the retina.

The term 'cytoid bodies' should be reserved for the histological finding of this phenomenon rather than the clinical presentation of cotton wool exudates. They occur as infarction of the nerve fibre layer in the retina where Wällerian degeneration of the neurons develops. Papilloedema may also be a prominent finding in these systemic inflammations.

Connective tissue diseases

Definition
- Systemic vasculitis with tissue disorders including arthralgias and arthritis

Presentation
- Iridocyclitis
- Scleritis
- Vitritis
- Retinitis
- Vasculitis
- Nongranulomatous

Investigation
- Antinuclear antibody
- Erythrocyte sedimentation rate
- Lupus anticoagulation
- Partial thromboplastin time
- Serum immune complexes (Raji)

Therapy
- Periocular corticosteroids
- Systemic corticosteroids
- Immunosuppressant agents (chlorambucil, cyclophosphamide)
- Cyclosporin

Complications
- Retinal ischaemia
- Chronic retinitis and vasculitis
- Nerve ischaemia
- Infarction of the retina

Prognosis
- Fair

Table 1.6   Connective tissue diseases.

2.
Endocrine Disorders

Table 2.1 Endocrine disorders: diabetes mellitus, hyperthyroidism, hypothyroidism.

DIABETES MELLITUS

A summary of endocrine disorders which affect the eye is presented in Table **2.1**. In the United States, diabetes mellitus is diagnosed by the ophthalmologist in one-third of cases because of the very characteristic signs in the fundus of the eye (**2.1–2.17**).

The earliest stages of retinopathy include the histological picture of closed capillaries, which are not seen ophthalmoscopically, but as the retinopathy becomes more severe, areas of capillary closure and nonperfusion become apparent. These are often marked by cotton wool spots (soft exudates), which are infarctions in the nerve fibre layer of the retina. These may fade or intensify over months. Microaneurysms and tortuous vessels are seen concurrently. Intraretinal microvascular abnormalities (IRMA) is a term that includes the dilated pre-existing capillaries or intraretinal new vessels, which have grown as a response to hypoxia in the retina. Haemorrhages accompany the exudation of proteinaceous material into the surrounding capillary spaces. Venous beading is a late accompaniment with blot haemorrhages in the retina. Together all these lesions are considered as nonproliferative diabetic retinopathy (NPDR). The vascular changes may become more severe or 'preproliferative,' leading to blindness. If capillary closure in retinal nonperfusion intensifies and becomes extensive over the retina, the ophthalmoscopic picture may be misleading and not represent the true severity of histological disease.

Intravenous fluorescein angiography, and more importantly now, indocyanine green angiography, will disclose a much more detailed picture of vessel closure and retinal tissue nonperfusion.

The appearance of new fragile blood vessels on the surface of the optic disc (neovascularization of the disc, NVD) or on the surface of the retina (neovascularization elsewhere, NVE) portends proliferative diabetic retinopathy (PDR), a more severe state. Usually the new vessels arise if not on the disc, then within 45° of the optic nerve head. These vessels are friable and tend to bleed easily and can therefore cause considerable damage in the vitreous and retina, leading to traction retinal detachment. While the natural history for these vessels is to increase and haemorrhage into the vitreous, they may also tend to regress. One of the principal mechanisms of visual loss in PDR is repeated vitreous haemorrhage leading to fibrous tissue formation and organization of the vitreous, and eventual traction retinal detachment.

The principal treatment of PDR is photocoagulation, which aims to induce regression of the new vessels, either on the disc or in the retina, eliminating the source of vitreous haemorrhage and inhibiting proliferation of fibrous tissue. There are many theories as to why this treatment works, but none has yet been proven. Panretinal photocoagulation is still the treatment of choice as promulgated by national studies, while direct treatment and focal treatment may also be used for a few or very specific focal manifestations of PDR. When severe vitreous haemorrhage, retinal distortion, or traction retinal detachment occurs despite full and prescribed photocoagulation, removal of the vitreous by vitrectomy surgery and tissue sectioning of fibrous bands is often recommended. Photocoagulation in the proximity of retinal traction fibrous bands may cause a worsening of traction retinal detachment due to contraction of these fibrous tissues and photocoagulation may be recommended only in conjunction with vitrectomy surgery, intraoperatively.

Macular oedema, even in NPDR, is still one of the leading causes of blindness in diabetes and 'grid' treatment has been advocated, scattering small burns except for within 500 μm of the centre of the macula.

It is not clear how grid treatment reduces oedema in the macula, but recent controlled studies have demonstrated a 50% reduction in moderate visual loss with this type of photocoagulation.

The incidence of diabetic retinopathy, especially PDR, is related to duration of the diabetes. Prevalence of PDR in patients aged 30 or older at diagnosis with a duration of 20 years was 25% in those taking insulin, and 5% in those not taking medication. The appearance of diabetic changes in the retina tends to occur 12–15 years after the onset of diagnosis in about 20% of all cases of diabetes.

Other mechanisms of blindness in diabetes include the following.
- Neovascular glaucoma caused by the growth of new blood vessels on the iris and in the anterior chamber angle. It is progressive and usually refractory to treatment.
- Chronic open-angle glaucoma, which is more common in diabetics than in the general population, but management of this type of intraocular pressure does not present more difficult problems.
- Cataract, which appears more commonly at a younger age in diabetic patients than in the general population.
- Diabetic patients who have a metabolic ketoacidosis are generally more vulnerable to infection and can develop infections of the extraocular tis-

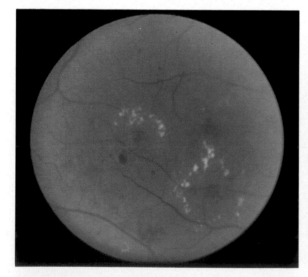

2.1 Retina demonstrating the small dot and blot haemorrhages and soft exudates that are characteristic of nonproliferative diabetic retinopathy, which is characterized by microaneurysm formation and leakage of blood and noncellular blood elements from incompetent capillary beds.

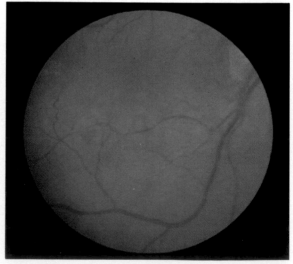

2.2 Minimal background diabetic retinopathy showing ophthalmoscopically evident macular oedema due to incompetent capillary beds in this patient. There is some tortuosity to the vessels.

sues and orbit from *Mucor* species, a fungus of the Phycomycetes class that causes a thrombosing arteritis and ischaemic necrosis in and around the orbit, the nose and the sinuses. The outcome may be fatal if not diagnosed and treated promptly.

Recent evidence suggests that very strict glycaemic control of patients with diabetes mellitus with divided doses more than twice a day will have a beneficial influence on the development of retinopathy, reducing its incidence by 25–50% compared to the control groups. Nephropathy is even more significantly reduced in these patients.

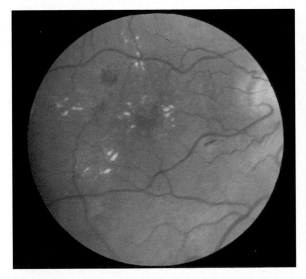

2.3 Leakage of noncellular proteinaceous elements produces retinal oedema as seen throughout the posterior pole of this patient. The hard exudates represent lipoprotein oedema residues, which are readily apparent throughout the posterior pole, as well as scattered dot and blot haemorrhages.

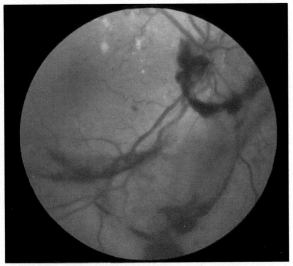

2.4 Proliferative diabetic retinopathy with new blood vessel formation at the optic disc evident by a subhyaloid haemorrhage which is spreading along the surface of the retina. This patient would be a candidate for panretinal photocoagulation laser therapy.

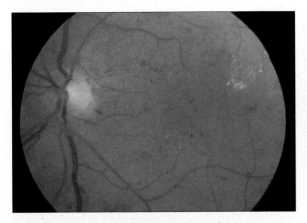

2.5 Scattered dot and blot haemorrhages throughout the fundus of this 26-year-old male with diabetes mellitus.

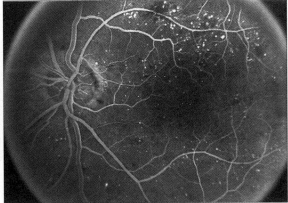

2.6 Fluorescein angiogram of patient in 2.5 demonstrating patchy retinal ischaemia from capillary closure, which is much more apparent with the fluorescein angiogram, focal areas of nonperfusion, exudation, and microaneurysm formation, forming what is called intraretinal microangiopathy (IRMA). Notice how much more obvious this is in the superior portion of the fundus on the angiogram than in the clinical photograph.

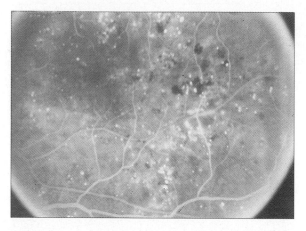

2.7 Late angiogram after venous filling demonstrating a large area of capillary nonperfusion superotemporally.

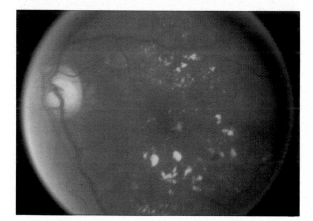

2.8 Hard waxy exudates in the retina represent lipoprotein residues from poor capillary bed circulation in a a 64-year-old white male with type 2 diabetes mellitus.

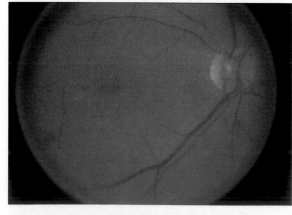

2.9 Neovascularization of the disc or early proliferative diabetic retinopathy, which marks this 31-year-old white female patient as a candidate for laser treatment.

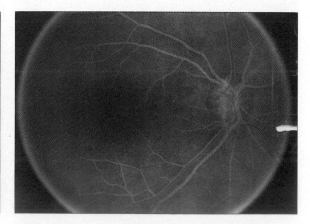

2.10 Early venous filling stage of fluorescein angiogram of the patient in 2.9 demonstrating the friable lacy neovascularization network protruding from the optic papillae and easily demarcated by angiography.

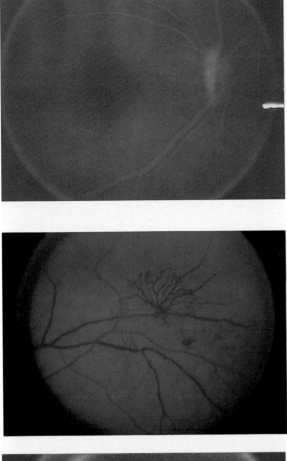

2.11 Late-phase angiogram demonstrating the full filling and leakage of the neovascularization on the disc of the patient in **2.9**.

2.12 Proliferative diabetic retinopathy represented as neovascularization elsewhere in a 27-year-old white male, demonstrating a friable lacy network in the retina superotemporal from the disc.

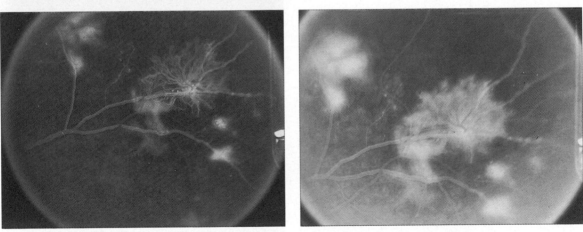

2.13 A venous filling stage of angiogram (left) demonstrating the full arborization network of the proliferative diabetic change classified as "neovascularization elsewhere" (NVE). **(right) Mid-phase angiogram** demonstrating the leakage from the friable vessels into the surrounding capillary bed and into the vitreous overlying the area. Note the other small areas of proliferative diabetic retinopathy (PDR), both supranasal and infratemporal, from the arborized NVE. Late-phase angiogram showing diffuse leakage from this neovascularization network now obscuring the original morphology of the friable vessels which composed it. Note the leakage into the vitreous even beyond the borders of the new blood vessels. While many patients with nonproliferative diabetic retinopathy (NPDR) will progress to PDR over time, some will not. Approximately 15% of patients with severe NPDR will develop moderately severe proliferative disease within 1 year. It is stated that 40% of all diabetic patients will develop PDR over a 15-year period.

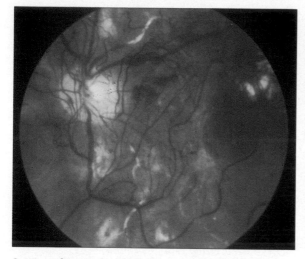

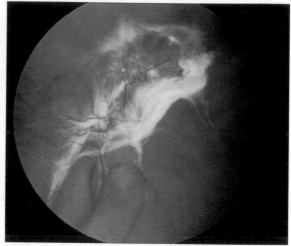

2.14 Advanced proliferative diabetic retinopathy with arborization of neovascular vessels emanating from the disc over the surface of the retina toward the macula, with early scar tissue formation in several foci.

2.15 A more advanced state of proliferative diabetic retinopathy classified as proliferans. Note the traction-induced elevation of the retina as it is pulled into the fibrous scar above it. The elevation of this scar tissue is complicated by the bridging bands of fibrovascular tissue, some of which have now been closed off by its own scarring, others of which are patent and would demonstrate moderate to advanced leakage on fluorescein angiography. This patient may be a candidate for vitrectomy surgery to relieve traction on the retina below this enlarging and progressing fibrovascular scar.

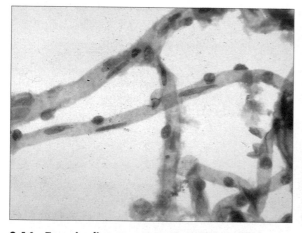

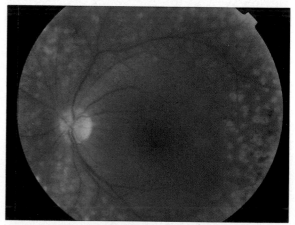

2.16 Trypsin digest preparation of the retina demonstrating profound loss of mural cells along the walls of the vessels in this capillary bed.

2.17 Posterior pole of patient with panretinal photocoagulation (PRP) demonstrating an optic nerve head free of neovascularization of the disc and a macula free of oedema and neovascularization elsewhere. Note the even ring of laser spots encompassing the peripheral retina. The Diabetic Retinopathy Study (DRS), a national cooperative research project, has demonstrated that photocoagulation can reduce the rate of visual loss by more than 50% in patients with proliferative diabetic retinopathy. Usually 1200–1800 50–100 μ burns are placed in treatment sessions; some patients respond readily to a relatively small amount of photocoagulation, while others may require repeated treatments to resolve neovascularization.

THYROID DYSFUNCTION

HYPERTHYROIDISM (GRAVES' DISEASE)

Hyperthyroidism frequently presents with ocular findings (**2.18–2.24**) before any systemic disease is diagnosed in the patient. The common triad of diffuse goitre, ophthalmopathy and dermopathy may be found. Thyroid adenoma, thyroid carcinoma, and hyperpituitarism may also cause hyperthyroidism and need to be ruled out as potentially life-threatening causes of hyperthyroidism.

The systemic signs and symptoms of hyperthyroidism include nervousness, irritability, fatigue, weight loss, emotional lability, heat intolerance, sweating, weakness, and palpitations, and may be explained on the basis of increased titres of thyroxine (T_4) and triiodothyronine (T_3). However, the ocular manifestations may occur in the absence of elevated T_4 and T_3 and include lid retraction, lagophthalmos, periorbital and conjunctival chemosis and oedema, restrictive extraocular myopathy, and proptosis. These findings are usually secondary to infiltrated extraocular muscles, which are engorged by a predominance of lymphoid cells. Enlarged episcleral vessels over the rectus muscle insertions may also be noted and can cause diplopia and even glaucoma due to the restriction of vascular engorgement of the recti.

Long-standing inflammation of the muscles leads to fibrosis, causing a lid retraction, lagophthalmos, and restrictions of the extraocular muscles. All of these findings may cause exposure with dry eye,

corneal abrasion, and recurrent corneal ulcers. Visual loss is usually due either to the problems of corneal exposure or compression of the optic nerve by the engorged rectus muscles, which become grossly enlarged and may be noted on magnetic resonance imaging or computerized tomography.

HYPOTHYROIDISM

When hypothyroidism occurs at birth, it results in developmental abnormalities, which has unfortunately been termed 'cretinism'. 'Myxoedema' refers to the severe form of hypothyroidism that results from deposition of mucopolysaccharides in the skin and other tissues in the later acquired disease.

Hypothyroidism usually begins insidiously and its symptoms include lethargy, constipation, cold intolerance, and, in females, menorrhagia. Motor weakness, loss of appetite, weight gain, dry skin, brittle hair, and the classical myxoedema of sparse hair and cool skin are accompaniments. In the classical condition, patients with myxoedema are said to have a dull expressionless face.

The ocular manifestations include loss of the temporal one-third to one-half of the eyelashes and brow. Conjunctival oedema and chemosis may be features along with blepharoptosis, nyctalopia, corneal oedema, keratoconus, strabismus, papilloedema, exophthalmos, cataracts, and even optic atrophy. The pathophysiological mechanisms for these ocular findings are not as straightforward as they are for the exposure problems due to the engorged rectus muscles (seen in hyperthyroidism).

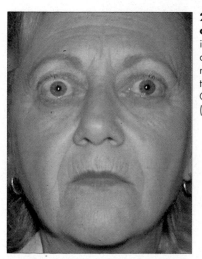

2.18 Thyroid ophthalmopathy in a patient demonstrating lid retraction as one of the earliest signs of Graves' disease (von Graefe's sign).

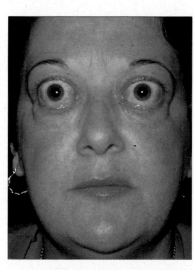

2.19 Note extreme lid retraction and 'stare' in patient with hyperthyroid exophthalmos. Note the scleral show on the inferior part of the eye on both sides.

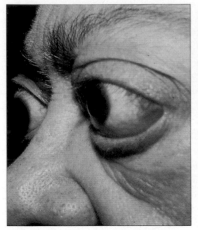

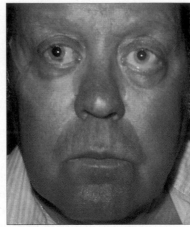

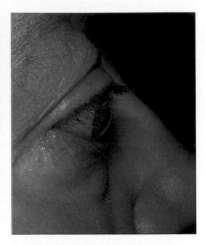

2.20 The same patient as in 2.19. Note the profound conjunctival and episcleral inflammation inferiorly in both eyes, which is a consequence of full daytime exposure.

2.21 Middle-aged male with thyroid exophthalmos, lid retraction, and corneal exposure in both eyes. Unlike the previous two patients, both lower and upper eyelids above the tarsus are engorged and swollen. This engorgement is similar to the extraocular muscle inflammation. Note the asymmetry to the eyelid retraction and bulbar exposure. While Graves' disease is usually bilateral, asymmetry is often the rule.

2.22 The same patient as in 2.21 in profile. Note how the profile emphasizes the lower palpebral and upper palpebral swelling and engorgement, almost making the patient's proptosis on frontal view look nonexistent.

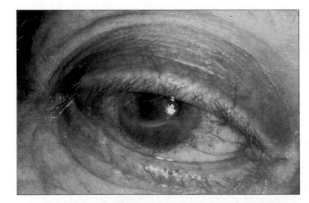

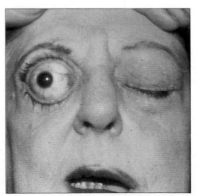

2.24 Extreme proptosis in the right eye of this patient with acute Graves' disease, with almost total lid retraction of the upper lid on the right side.

2.23 Intensely inflamed thyroid exophthalmic eye with corneal exposure and early corneal ulcer formation with dehiscence of the epithelium.

PITUITARY DISORDERS

Pituitary adenomas and other mass-occupying lesions forming suprasellar masses must be at least 10 mm in size before they can compress the chiasm and interrupt blood flow (**2.25**). When this occurs, they produce the classical bitemporal hemianopia. Post-fixed chiasms may demonstrate ipsilateral optic nerve compression, whereas pre-fixed chiasms produce an incongruous contralateral homonymous hemianopia with a subtle contralateral afferent pupillary defect when this is compromised. The ocular sign of an optic nerve compression is usually optic atrophy and the temporal disc may be pale due to atrophy of the papillomacular fibres. In optic track compression, the characteristic 'bow tie' atrophy in the contralateral eye is usually less than the more diffuse atrophy in the ipsilateral eye. Very rarely, papilloedema may predate the actual optic atrophy.

About one-third of patients with acromegaly have adenomas that hypersecrete both growth hormone and prolactin and may have symptoms of hyperprolactinemia.

The usual treatment for pituitary adenomas and other paracellular lesions that cause visual abnormalities is neurosurgical excision, but radiation may be used. Prolactinomas and other endocrine-secreting neoplasms such as a somatotrophic adenoma, may respond to long-acting chemical hormone treatment.

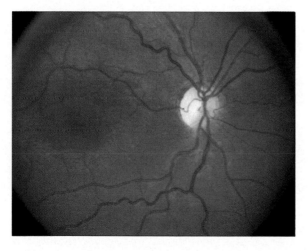

2.25 Profound temporal optic atrophy in a 10-year-old white male with a pituitary adenoma compressing the optic chiasma leading to this optic atrophy and loss of vision. Such tumours are usually in the anterior lobe of the pituitary and may also invade adjacent cavernous sinus, leading to compromise of the third, fourth and sixth cranial nerves and causing ophthalmoplegia.

3.
Vascular Disorders

Many pathological features associated with systemic vascular disorders such as hypertension, congenital heart disease, and pulmonary difficulties can be observed directly. Similarly, retinal vascular accidents, either arterial or venous, may reflect systemic disorders such as emboli arising from the heart or large blood vessels or from systemic afflictions such as exogenous intravenous drug abuse.

SYSTEMIC HYPERTENSION

Systemic hypertension may be reflected in the ocular fundus (**3.1–3.3**) in terms of irregularities in arteriolar calibre, tortuosity of the retinal arterioles, and changes at the arteriovenous crossings. Progressive and more severe hypertensive changes include generalized arteriolar narrowing with various degrees of

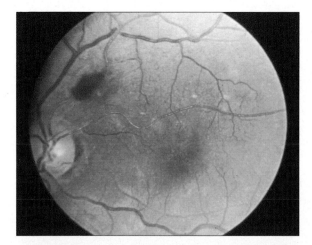

3.1 A 54-year-old male patient with moderately severe systemic hypertension. Note the retinal arterioles are attenuated and irregular and the flame-shaped haemorrhage superotemporal to the disc with a white centre. Soft exudates are present demonstrating some infarction of the nerve fibre layer.

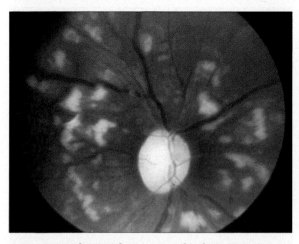

3.2 Very advanced renovascular hypertensive changes in the fundus of a 41-year-old African–American male demonstrating cotton wool exudation extensively over the surface of the retina, indicating infarction of the nerve fibre layer, and a profound end-stage optic atrophy.

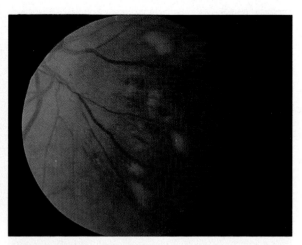

3.3 A 48-year-old white female with hypertensive retinopathy peripherally of cotton wool exudation.

Vascular disorders

Definition
- Retinal artery or vein occlusion (branch or central), haematological disorders

Presentation
- Decreased vision
- Haemorrhage, exudate, or ischaemic change in the retina
- Pain (neovascular glaucoma)

Investigation
- Hypertension
- Cardiovascular disease
- Haematological: leukaemia, lymphoma, anaemia

Therapy
- Treat underlying disease
- Laser treatment of retina

Complications
- Cystoid macular oedema
- Neovascular glaucoma
- Central nervous system (cerebrovascular accident – thrombosis or haemorrhage)
- Myocardial infarction

Prognosis
- Variable

Table 3.1 Vascular disorders.

retinal ischaemia, which is manifest as cotton wool exudation or infarction of the nerve fibre layer of the retina, haemorrhages, retinal oedema, and even, in late cases, papilloedema.

RETINAL ARTERIAL OCCLUSIVE DISEASE

Retinal arterial occlusive disease can be seen in many systemic disorders (**3.4–3.26, Table 3.1**) including:
- Ocular ischaemic syndrome.
- Carotid artery obstruction.
- Calcification with plaque.
- Ophthalmic artery obstruction.
- Central retinal artery obstruction (CRAO), which may be due to intraluminal thrombosis.
- Haemorrhage under or from an arteriosclerotic plaque.
- Spasm.
- Vasculitis.
- Dissecting aneurysm.
- Hypertensive arteriolar necrosis.
- Circulatory collapse.

Associated diseases that contribute to such an occlusive process include:
- Arterial hypertension.
- Diabetes mellitus (25% of people with CRAO have an associated diabetes mellitus, whereas the incidence for an age-matched group is less than 10%).
- Carotid arteriosclerosis with cardiac valvular disease.

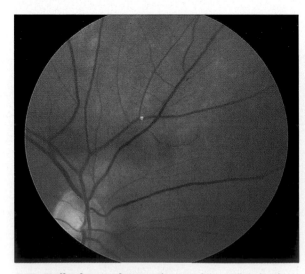

3.4 Hollenhorst plaque. This is a shiny, yellow lipid embolism lodged in a bifurcation of a retinal arteriole superotemporally. It originated from an atheromatous plaque in a carotid artery. Note that there is no attendant infarction with this asymptomatic embolism.

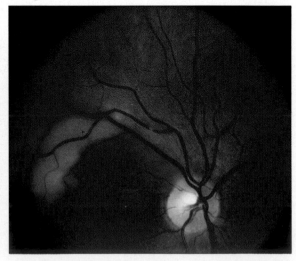

3.5 Superotemporal branch artery occlusion secondary to Hollenhorst plaque seen as a glistening yellow lipid embolism.

- Collagen vascular disorders, including giant cell arteritis as well as the other collagenoses.
- Trauma.
- Coagulopathies, which include sickling haemoglobinopathies such as sickle trait, especially when the intraocular pressure is above normal.

People with lupus anticoagulants, antibodies to the IgM or IgG class, have a prolonged partial thromboplastin time. This may also lead to branch retinal artery obstruction or even a cilioretinal artery obstruction and be a consequence of any of the systemic diseases listed above.

Other rare systemic conditions that may contribute to CRAO include radiological studies such as lymphangiography, carotid angiography, and ventriculography, retrobulbar injections, orbital fracture, general anaesthesia, drug- or alcohol-induced stupor, homocystinuria, oral contraceptives, pregnancy, other platelet factor abnormalities, Fabry's disease, optic neuritis, radiation retinopathy, and migraine.

Emboli of cardiac origin may be either secondary to rheumatic heart disease, mitral valve disorders, mural thrombus, or myxoma of the heart. The calcified emboli from rheumatic valves tend to be larger and more white in appearance than cholesterol emboli. Because of their greater size, they have an increased tendency to cause clinically apparent arterial obstruction, glisten when seen in the ocular fundus, and look to be larger than the lumen they are obstructing. Calcific emboli are thought to arise from the aortic valve in particular. Glistening yellow cholesterol emboli, also known as Hollenhorst plaques, most often originate from arteriosclerotic carotid artery intraluminal plaque.

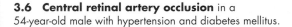

3.6 Central retinal artery occlusion in a 54-year-old male with hypertension and diabetes mellitus.

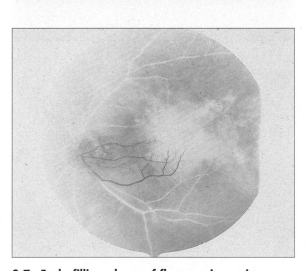

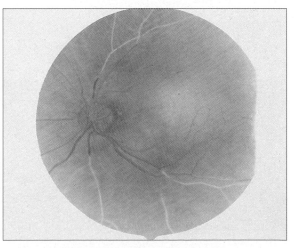

3.7 Early-filling phase of fluorescein angiogram of patient in **3.5** demonstrating ischaemia and infarction of the macula due to cilioretinal artery occlusion.

3.8 Late-phase angiogram demonstrating very late filling of the arterioles and infarcted macula.

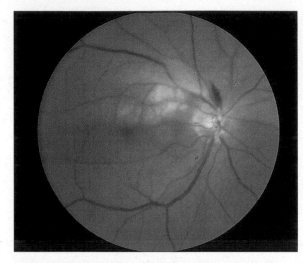

3.9 A 62-year-old male with superotemporal branch artery occlusion and infarction of the underlying retina. Note the chalky white calcific embolism just inferior to the flame-shaped haemorrhage.

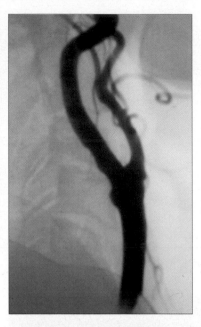

3.10 Carotid angiogram demonstrating moth-eaten indentation at the location of a calcified plaque, which was throwing emboli into the retina and central nervous system.

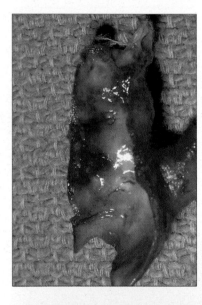

3.11 Excised section of carotid artery demonstrating the necrotic moth-eaten calcified plaque. Notice that it is small enough not to obliterate the lumen of this vessel, but has enough calcific necrosis to be throwing off multiple small embolic pieces.

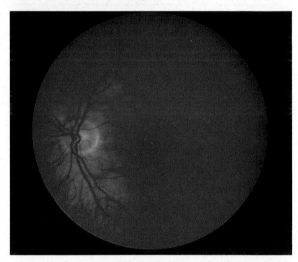

3.12 Hollenhorst plaque inferotemporal to the macula of this patient without visual symptoms.

3.13 Fluorescein angiogram of a patient with a central retinal artery occlusion. Note the lack of arteriole filling by 16.5 seconds.

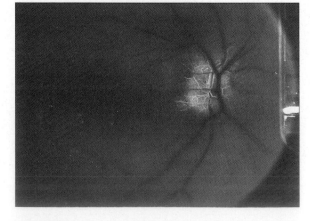

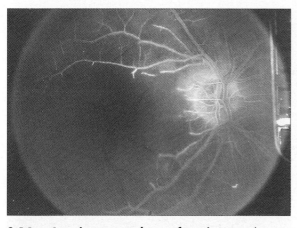

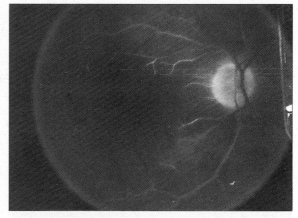

3.14a Arteriovenous phase of angiogram showing ischaemic macula and posterior pole due to central artery occlusion.

3.14b Late-phase angiogram at 398 seconds still shows some sluggish flow in the arterioles and leakage of the optic nerve head.

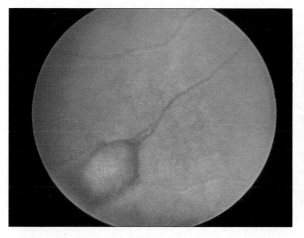

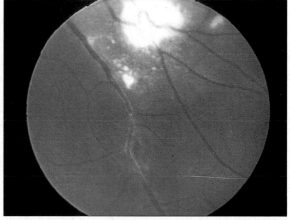

3.15 A 19-year-old African–American male with sickle cell retinopathy demonstrating a pale pink retinal haemorrhage with a tortuous feeder vessel. This is the classic 'salmon' patch of sickle cell retinopathy due to haemorrhage involving the deep layers of the retina.

3.16 A 26-year-old African–American female with sickle cell disease demonstrating a white retinal pigment epithelial disturbance secondary to what was pigment hyperplasia with iridescent granules known as a 'sun burst' sign, which is due to haemorrhage leaving a small retinoschisis cavity causing the iridescent appearance. These are haemorrhages in the deep layers of the retina.

3.17 An 11-year-old African–American male with sickle cell disease demonstrating an intensely red salmon patch secondary to deep retinal haemorrhage and infarction.

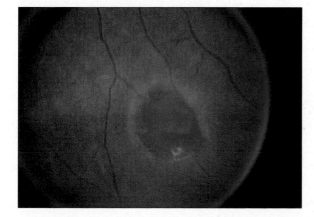

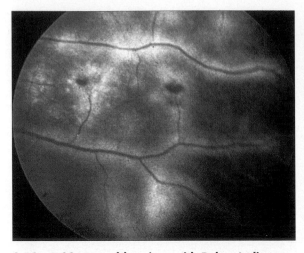

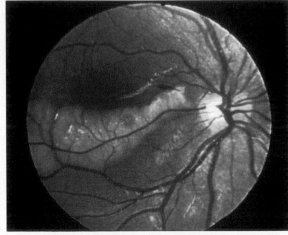

3.18 A 22-year-old patient with Behçet's disease demonstrating a very marked vasculitis of both the arteriolar and venular tree.

3.19 Central retinal artery occlusion infarcting one-half of the macula providing this dramatic picture of hemimacular ischaemia.

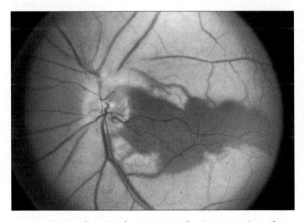

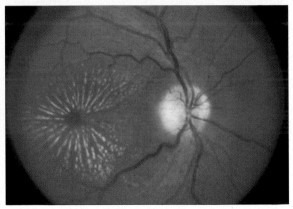

3.20 Central retinal artery occlusion sparing the ciliioretinal artery, which still feeds and nourishes the macula, preserving central vision while peripheral vision is obliterated. Contrast this to the previous picture of central retinal artery occlusion, which is its mirror image in reverse.

3.21 Macular star and optic pallor in a patient with resolved stigmata of central retinal artery occlusion, but the macula is still extremely oedematous, giving rise to this radiating pattern of oedema along the nerve fibres.

3.22 Infratemporal branch artery occlusion in a patient with a very obvious glistening white calcific embolism in the inferior aspect of the optic nerve head.

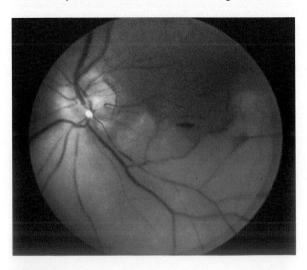

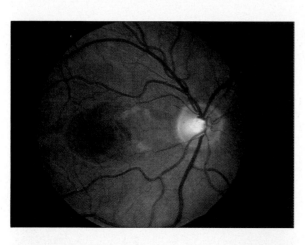

3.23 A 27-year-old white male with unexplained cilioretinal artery occlusion. This patient was worked-up for connective tissue disease and found not to have one.

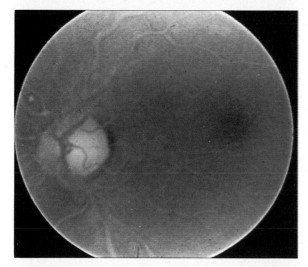

3.24 A 28-year-old African–American male with lipaemia retinalis.

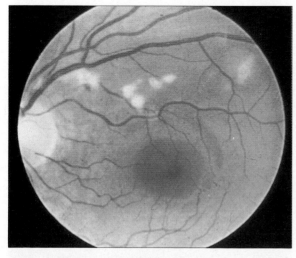

3.25 A 22-year-old white male with fat emboli along the superotemporal arcades from massive leg fractures in an automobile accident.

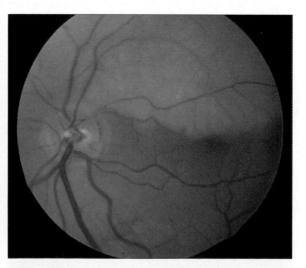

3.26 Dramatic fundal picture showing hemiretinal ischaemia superiorly from branch artery occlusion. Note the large white embolism situated centrally in the optic papilla obstructing the superior artery before it bifurcates into the temporal and nasal branches.

RETINAL VEIN OCCLUSION

Central retinal vein occlusion usually results in profound visual loss due to thrombosis of the central retinal vein (**3.27– 3.36**). Hemicentral retinal vein thrombosis is usually an anatomical variant of the central vein thrombus, while branch retinal vein occlusion usually involves just one of the tributaries of the central retinal vein.

The process causing thrombus formation in the central retinal vein occurs through either external compression with primary thrombus formation due to venous stasis in that vessel or degenerative or inflammatory disorders of the vein itself, some of which are due to a vasculitis at the arteriovenous juncture compressing the venule before the arteriole is closed. The systemic collagenoses and giant cell arteritis are often noted to do this.

Arteriosclerosis occurring at the lamina cribrosa where the intraluminal pressure of the vein decreases makes it especially vulnerable to collapse at this anatomical location. Arteriosclerosis is the most

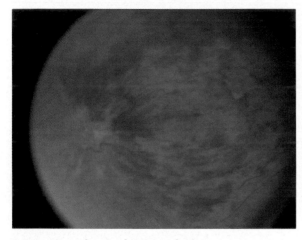

3.27 Central retinal vein occlusion in a 56-year-old patient with arteriosclerotic cardiovascular disease. Note the multiple haemorrhages scattered over the retina obscuring the dilated retinal veins. The optic disc is also swollen.

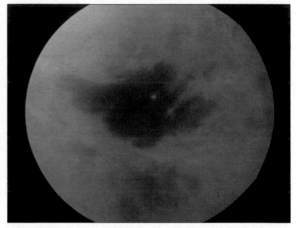

3.28 A 43-year-old white male with infratemporal vein occlusion demonstrated as a finite focus of haemorrhage in the retina.

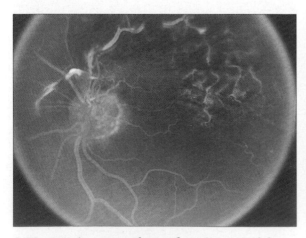

3.29 Arteriovenous phase of angiogram of the patient in 3.28. Note the overlying obscuration of fluorescein due to the haemorrhage and the beaded temporal branch vein where obstruction has occurred.

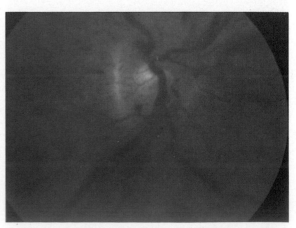

3.30 A 40-year-old patient with swelling of the optic nerve secondary to surrounding central retinal vein obstruction.

common factor in this disorder, but papilloedema can also lead to increased pressure within the optic nerve sheath and thereby compromise the central retinal vein lumen.

Ophthalmopathy due to thyroid disease, orbital tumour and abscess, cavernous sinus thrombosis, or retrobulbar injections with intranerve sheath compression can also cause and precipitate a central retinal vein occlusion.

Retinal vein occlusion may also result from a hyperviscosity syndrome such as hypergammaglobulinaemia, paraproteinaemia, hyperfibrinogenaemia, cryofibrinogenaemia and the blood dyscrasias of leukaemia, sickle cell disease, polycythaemia vera, and others. It is to be noted that systemic diseases such as malignancies 'with peripheral vascular effects,' paraproteinaemia, nephrotic syndrome, chronic obstructive pulmonary disease and Behçet's disease may all be associated with an elevated blood viscosity and may lead to central retinal vein occlusion on a hyperviscosity basis.

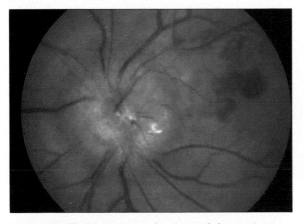

3.31 Papilloedematous changes of the optic nerve head with macular haemorrhage in a patient with pseudotumor cerebri, which was misdiagnosed as a central retinal vein occlusion.

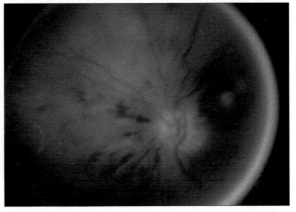

3.32 A 59-year-old white female with profound retinal oedema and striated haemorrhages due to central retinal vein occlusion.

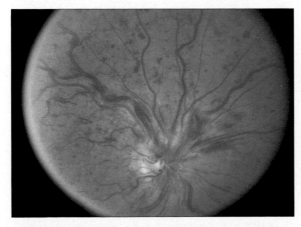

3.33 A central retinal vein occlusion that has partially resorbed leaving various streaks and dot haemorrhages in a retina with a swollen optic nerve head.

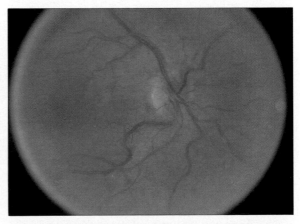

3.34 Impending central retinal vein occlusion in a 60-year-old white male showing tortuous vessels, but no dot or blot haemorrhages in the retina as yet. This patient had atherosclerotic cardiovascular disease and later developed a full-blown central retinal vein occlusion 3 months later.

RETINAL VASCULITIS

Retinal vasculitis associated with the collagenoses and demonstrated by cotton wool exudation or infarction of the nerve fibre layer and haemorrhage in the retina in conjunction with vasculitic changes, would include polyarteritis nodosum, Wegener's granulomatosis, systemic lupus erythematosus, Whipple's disease, Behçet's disease, sarcoidosis, multiple sclerosis, Crohn's disease, polychondritis, and very occasionally, ankylosing spondylitis and the other HLA B27-positive arthritides (**3.37–3.39**). While all the above-mentioned conditions may cause vasculitis, it is to be noted that sarcoidosis has a predilection to cause periphlebitis with venous sheathing, more prominent inflammation of vessels

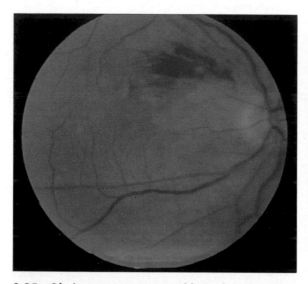

3.35 Obvious superotemporal branch vein occlusion in a patient with systemic hypertension.

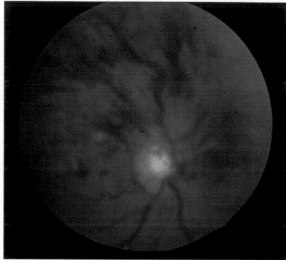

3.36 A 65-year-old African–American female with branch vein occlusion superotemporally showing soft exudates of infarction of the nerve fibre layer along with the intraretinal haemorrhage.

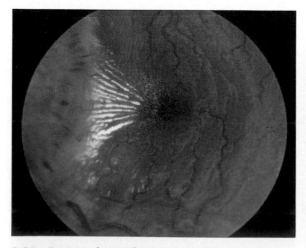

3.37 Temporal macular 'star' formation in a young patient with lupus erythematosus and renal hypertension with infarction and disorganization of the retina temporal to the macula.

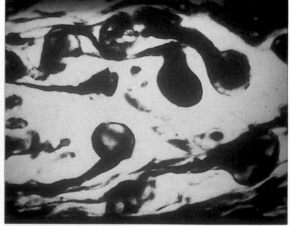

3.38 'Cytoid' bodies with Hortega stain of the retinal nerve fibre layer. Note the rolled-up 'lollipop' nerve endings, which represent Wallerian degeneration of the nerve fibres along its peripheral axons rolling up towards its origin. These infarctions with Wallerian degeneration of the neurons are typically seen in connective tissue disorders as well as in severe hypertensive retinopathy.

on the venular side than on the arteriolar side, and an association with choroidal granulomas and neovascularization in the retina.

Polyarteritis nodosa, systemic lupus erythematosus and Behçet's disease are multisystem disorders that can affect all coats of the eye, and in addition to their hallmark of obliterative vasculitis in the retina, cause a panuveitis.

HAEMATOPOIETIC AND LYMPHORETICULAR DISORDERS

The abnormalities in the number and structure of the blood cells changes the blood viscosity and may be associated with numerous ocular manifestations (**3.40–3.65**) including a coagulative arteriolar or venular obstruction, haemorrhages in the retina, Roth's

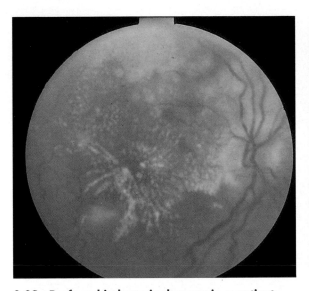

3.39 Profound ischaemic changes in a patient with connective tissue disease demonstrating a macular star formation and retinal ischaemia for two-thirds of the retina.

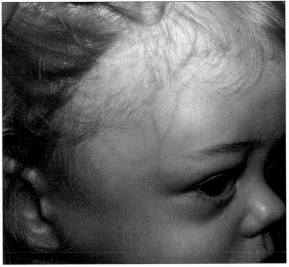

3.40 A 28-month-old white female with swollen periorbital region, which was classically termed 'chloroma' of myelogenous leukaemic infiltrate in and around the orbit.

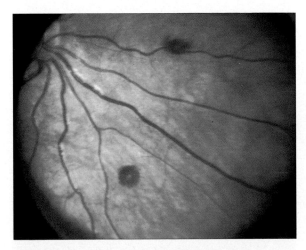

3.41 Roth spot in the retina of the patient in 3.40, which demonstrates a round red haemorrhage surrounding a central focus of myelogenous cells. Roth spots are also seen in subacute bacterial endocarditis as well as other infections in the eye and myelogenous leukaemia.

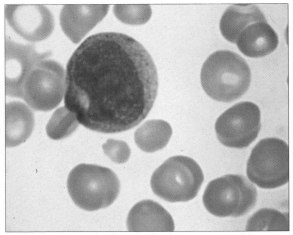

3.42 Peripheral blood of the patient in 3.40 showing Auer rod in a myelogenous cell.

spots, and even papillitis and papilloedema. Anaemia, leukaemia, lymphoma, sickle cell disease, and lymphoreticular neoplasms all have ocular manifestations. Roth's spots result from septic emboli in patients with subacute bacterial endocarditis and are oval or elongated haemorrhages with a white centre, which contains inflammatory cells as well as the septic material, either particulate or infectious. Roth's spots are not pathognomonic of bacterial endocarditis. They are also found in myelogenous leukaemia, anaemia, and fungal retinitis, and as such represent a valuable diagnostic sign.

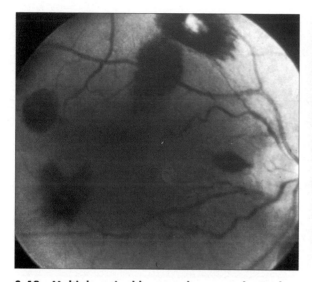

3.43 Multiple retinal haemorrhages and a Roth spot in a 34-year-old patient with acute myelogenous leukaemia.

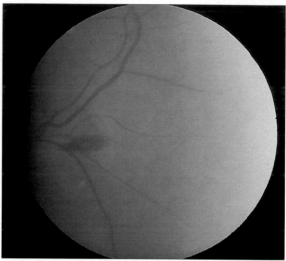

3.44 Flame-shaped haemorrhage, actually a Roth spot with a white centre, which was the only clinical finding to indicate that this patient had acute myelogenous leukaemia diagnosed on bone marrow aspiration.

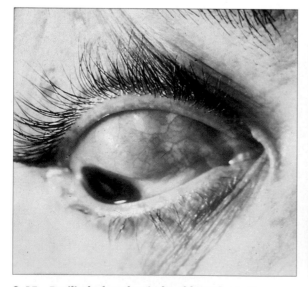

3.45 Perilimbal and episcleral lymphomatous infiltration in a patient.

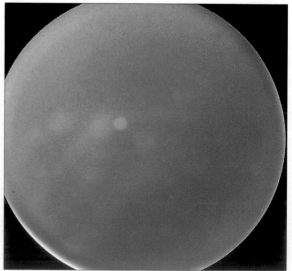

3.46 Vitreous clouding and subretinal infiltration in a patient with large cell lymphoma (reticulum cell sarcoma).

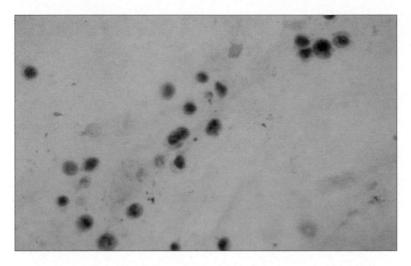

3.47 Vitreous aspirate showing neoplastic B cells in a patient with large cell lymphoma.

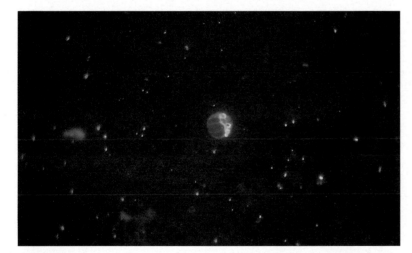

3.48 Vitreous stain for light chains demonstrating the monoclonal basis of the B-cell infiltrate in the vitreous and subretinal location. If only lambda or gamma light chains show (one stains with rhodamine, one stains with fluorescein), this indicates monoclonality.

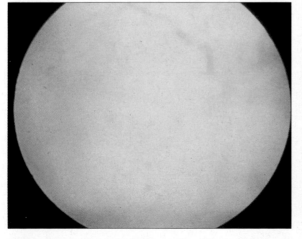

3.49 Dense vitreous infiltrate in a 62-year-old patient with B-cell lymphoma infiltration to the eye.

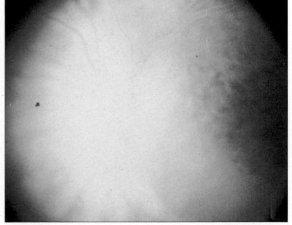

3.50 Fluorescein angiogram of the patient in 3.49 demonstrating obscuration by vitreous infiltration and accumulation of subretinal and optic nerve head infiltration by B-cell lymphoma.

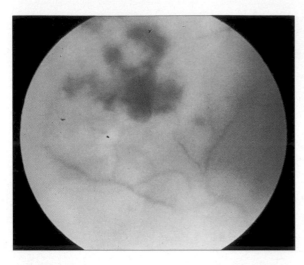

3.51 Haemorrhagic necrotic retina, which looks like a cytomegalovirus retinitis, but is in fact subretinal infiltration of B-cell lymphoma in a 72-year-old patient.

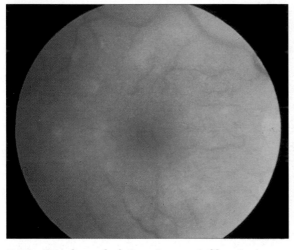

3.52 Macula underlying vitreous infiltration demonstrating small focal infiltrates of B-cell lymphoma in an 82-year-old patient with 'reticulum cell sarcoma'.

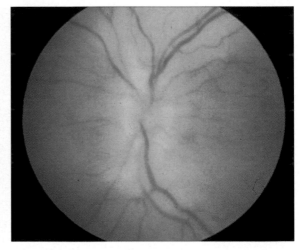

3.53 Optic nerve head of the patient in 3.52 showing optic nerve swelling from a B-cell lymphoma.

3.54 Macula of the fellow eye of patient in 3.52 showing very diffuse mottling of the retinal pigment epithelium.

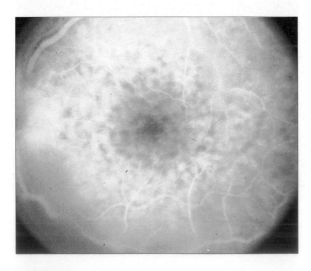

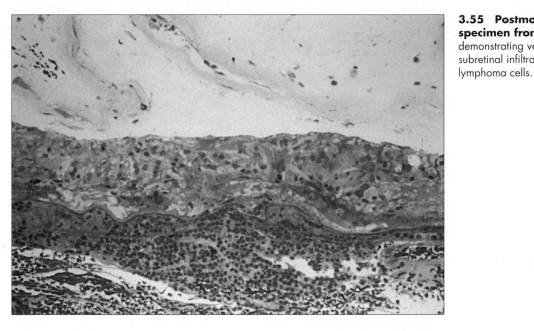

3.55 Postmortem specimen from retina demonstrating very marked subretinal infiltration with lymphoma cells.

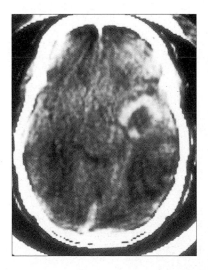

3.56 CAT scan of patient showing large focal brain tumour termed 'microgliomatosis' in patient with B-cell lymphoma or reticulum cell sarcoma.

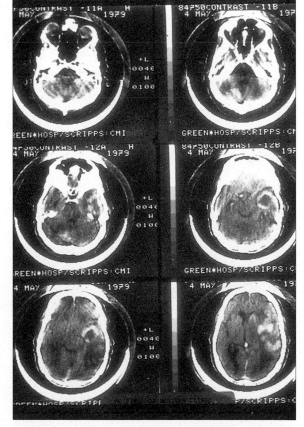

3.57 Several CAT scan views of the patient in 3.56 demonstrating the large evolving brain tumour of reticulum cell sarcoma.

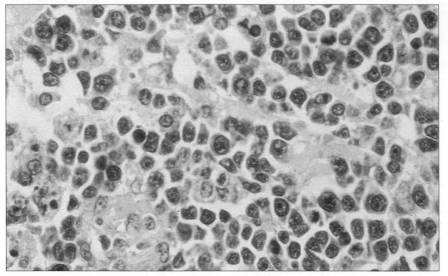

3.58 Brain biopsy of patient in 3.56 demonstrating diffuse lymphomatous infiltration of white matter tissue.

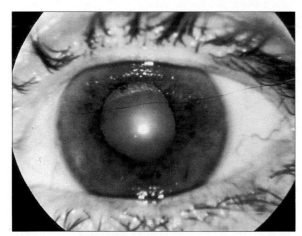

3.59 Intense vitreous infiltration of patient with chronic lymphocytic leukaemia manifesting as 'Richter syndrome,' which shows the multipotentiality of B-cell lymphoma to change along different stem cell lines.

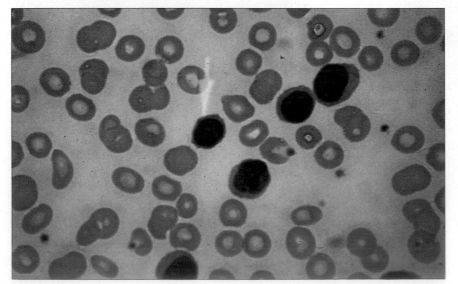

3.60 Peripheral blood of patient with chronic lymphocytic leukaemia demonstrating the abnormal neoplastic cells.

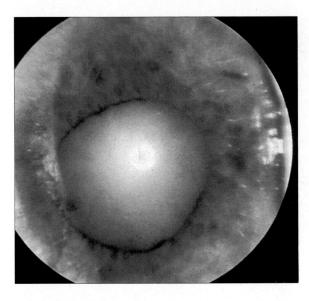

3.61   Higher magnification photograph of the intense vitreous inflammation in the patient in 3.60, which simulates a 'reticulum cell sarcoma,' but in fact is chronic lymphocytic leukaemia filling the vitreous, simulating a cataract at the slit lamp.

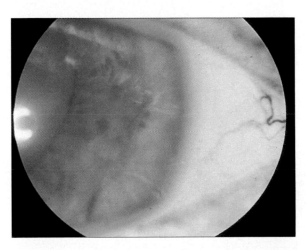

3.62   Note the peripheral iris in the patient in 3.60 demonstrating infiltration of the uveal tissue with leukaemia cells.

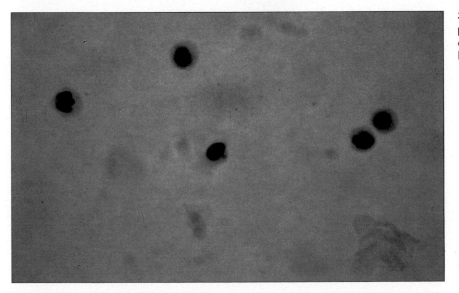

3.63   Vitreous of the patient in 3.60 showing chronic lymphocytic leukaemia cells.

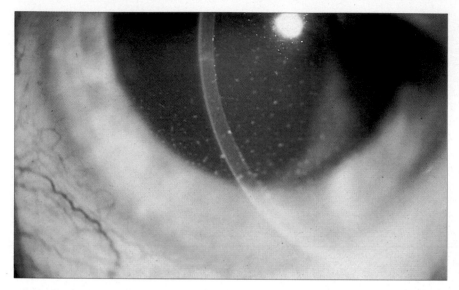

3.64 A 62-year-old white male with large cell lymphoma infiltration in the vitreous and choroid who has keratic precipitates and a profound anterior chamber cellular reaction, which is said to be rare or nonexistent in large cell lymphoma infiltration of the eye.

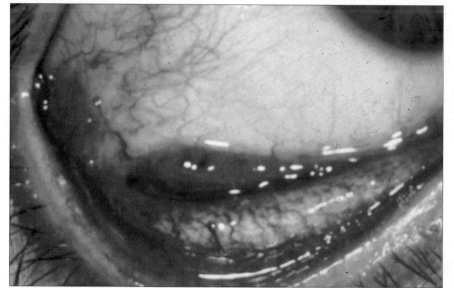

3.65 Large cell lymphomatous infiltration of periorbital tissues inferiorly with surrounding episcleritis and conjunctival erythema.

4.
Tumours

The most common malignant disorders of the eye are malignant melanoma in adults, metastatic cancers to the eye, and adnexa retinoblastoma in infants (**Table 4.1**). Retinoblastoma spreads by vascular routes to the long bones, usually after involving the optic nerve. Malignant melanoma metastasizes to the liver.

METASTATIC TUMOURS

Metastatic tumours (**4.1–4.9**) form a relatively small proportion of the cancers treated by ophthalmologists or oncologists, but are often the most serious because they represent metastatic spread through

Ocular tumours

Definition
- Neoplasms, primary or secondary to the eye: metastasis, melanoma, retinoblastoma, haemangioma of choroid, others (B cell lymphoma, benign choristomas, hamartomas)

Presentation
- Leukocoria (retinoblastoma)
- Decreased vision
- Retinal detachment: solid or rhegmatogenous
- Glaucoma

Investigation
- Magnetic resonance imaging
- Computerized axial tomography
- Ultrasound of eye
- Fluorescein angiogram
- Carcino-embryonic antigen (CEA)
- Other tumour-specific antigens (metastasis)
- Anti-melanoma antibodies

Therapy
- Variable
- Radiation
- Chemotherapy
- Laser
- Enucleation
- Evisceration

Complications
- Glaucoma
- Uveitis
- Retinal detachment
- Loss of eye
- Loss of life

Prognosis
- Variable

Table 4.1 Ocular tumours.
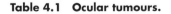

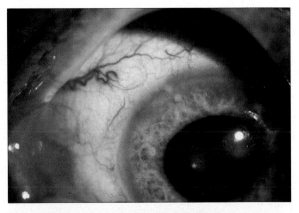

4.1 Peripheral iris lesion of pink fleshy metastasis from lung carcinoma.

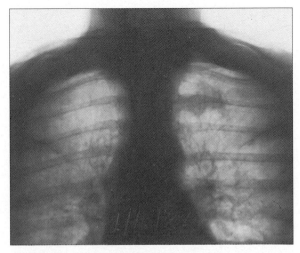

4.2 Chest radiograph of the patient in 4.1 demonstrating large apical carcinoma of the lung that had metastasized to the eye.

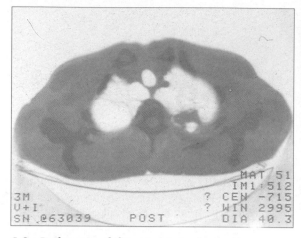

4.3 Body scan of thorax showing large apic carcinoma of the lung in the patient in **4.1**.

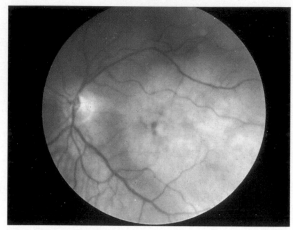

4.4 A 44-year-old white female with metastatic breast cancer to the posterior pole manifesting as a large 'mesa-shaped' infiltration in the choroid.

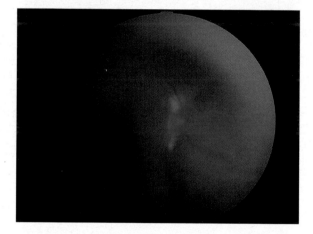

4.5 Fundus photograph showing adenocarcinoma of the lung metastatic to the choroid.

4.6 Arteriogram of lung demonstrating the fibrotic and vascular nature of this tumour.

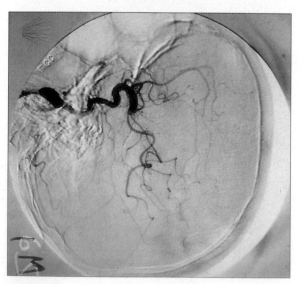

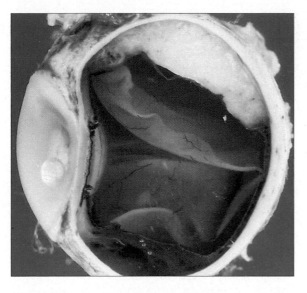

4.7 Gross anatomical specimen of patient with metastatic adenocarcinoma to the choroid.

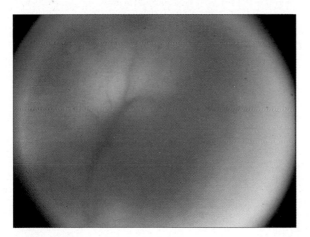

4.8 Typical presentation of vitritis and subretinal infiltration of large cell lymphoma in a patient with 'reticulum cell sarcoma' or non Hodgkin's B-cell lymphoma.

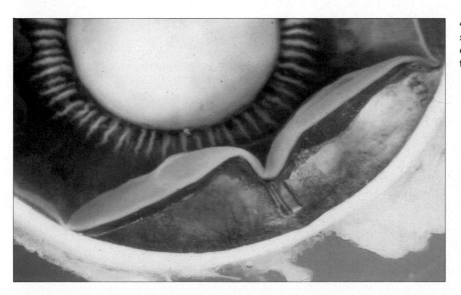

4.9 Gross specimen showing renal cell carcinoma metastatic to the ciliary body.

the body and to the eye. Carcinoma of the breast is the most common metastasizing systemic cancer to the eye, while lung cancer accounts for the majority of metastases to the eye in men. While cancer of the prostate has a tendency to metastasize to orbital bones, it rarely spreads to the intraocular tissues. Other tumours that occasionally metastasize to the eye and adnexa include carcinoma of the gastrointestinal tract (especially adenocarcinoma of the colon), renal cell carcinoma, thyroid carcinoma, carcinoid tumour and cutaneous malignant melanoma. Lymphoid tumours and leukaemias are discussed in a separate chapter. The vast majority of ocular metastases occur in adults, while lesions of neuroblastoma or Ewing's bone cancer can present in the ocular tissues and adnexa in children.

Tumours that metastasize to the intraocular structures usually involve the uveal tract, but most commonly occur in the posterior pole of the eye. Unlike malignant melanoma, which breaks through Bruch's membrane and usually forms a mushroom-shaped tumour, these tumours tend to form a table or mesa with identifiable edges and although elevated, are usually flattened on their top. This can be discerned both by clinical ophthalmoscopy and by ultrasound examination. Tumours metastatic to the retina itself, the optic nerve and the vitreous are comparatively rare, although reticulum cell sarcoma or large cell lymphoma has been noted to infiltrate the vitreous exclusively.

RETINOBLASTOMA

The median age of patients presenting with retinoblastoma (**4.10–4.14**), which is an autosomal recessively inherited cancer arising from the retina itself, is 18 months. It is often bilateral in the inherited familial form, but tends to be unilateral in sporadic cases. Its most prominent ocular sign is leukocoria, but may

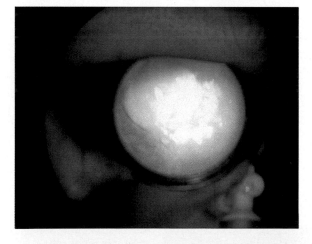

4.10 Fundus appearance of large fungating white retinoblastoma in a 2-year-old infant.

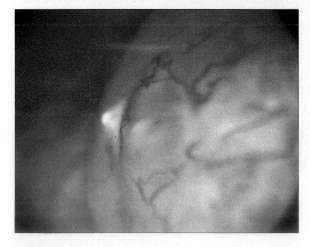

4.11 Atypical retinoblastoma because it appeared in an 18-year-old white male.

be noted as small peripheral tumours not seen with direct ophthalmoscopy. Any youngster presenting with esotropia should therefore have a dilated indi-rect ophthalmoscopic examination to exclude retino-blastoma or any other lesion that can cause blindness in the posterior pole.

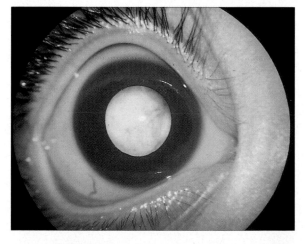

4.12 Gross specimen of the patient in 4.11 showing retinoblastoma arising from the retina.

4.13 A 9-month-old white female with retinoblastoma filling up the entire inside of the right eye.

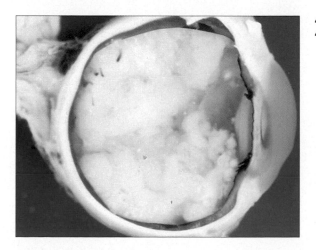

4.14 Gross anatomical specimen of the patient in 4.13

MALIGNANT MELANOMA

Malignant melanoma (**4.15–4.28**) can be seen in any age group, although usually it is more common after the age of 40. While iris melanomas are now considered almost exclusively in the benign category, and indeed although they may seem to grow, it is very rare for them to metastasize and be considered truly malignant. However, care is needed to eliminate the possibility of a ciliary body melanoma that has extended into the iris through the angle and which may be mistaken for a sole iris lesion. Careful dilation and ultrasonography of the eye, as well as scleral depression with indirect ophthalmoscopy, needs to be performed to rule out extension from a ciliary body melanoma. Ciliary body melanoma may also present as a 'ring' melanoma, growing in a 360° circumferential expansion, rather than an anterior–posterior fashion. These may be very malignant, having already metastasized to the liver by the time of recognition.

Choroidal malignant melanoma is still the most common intraocular malignancy met in practice other than a metastatic lesion to the eye. It may grow very slowly, and careful diagnosis may justify a period of observation. More than half of the malignant melanomas in the choroid are amelanotic and do not have the usual brown or grey appearance and may have orange patches of lipofuscin and ageing change in the retinal pigment epithelium overlying them. These usually grow in a collar button or mushroom cap shape, breaking through Bruch's membrane and extending out. Usually, after the 'collar-stud' growth, vessels may be seen coursing through the substance around the surface of the malignant melanoma. Its typical shape may be confirmed by ultrasonography with a classical appearance of choroidal excavation.

Extrascleral extension when it occurs on the globe itself is a sign of a poor prognosis and often represents early liver metastasis.

An eye with an insidious loss of vision with rubeosis of the iris and secondary glaucoma should be suspected of harbouring a malignant melanoma until proven otherwise, and this may be easily demonstrated by ultrasonography when the media is sufficiently opaque to preclude visualization into the eye.

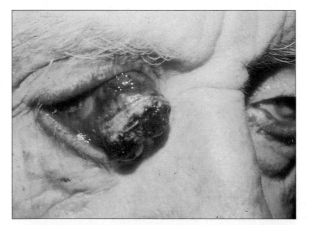

4.15 A 63-year-old male with malignant melanoma of the choroid extruding through ocular contents.

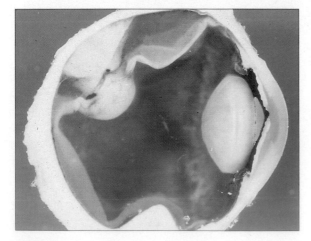

4.16 Typical mushroom-shaped amelanotic malignant melanoma of the choroid breaking through Bruch's membrane giving this classical and typical histological appearance.

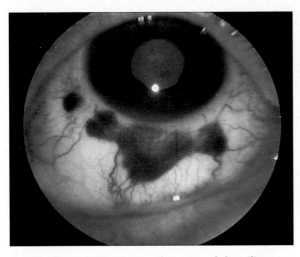

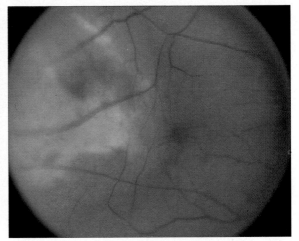

4.17 'Ring' malignant melanoma of the ciliary body infiltrating around the limbus. Classically, this tumour infiltrates for 360°.

4.18 Classical picture of choroidal malignant melanoma in its mushroom shape breaking through Bruch's membrane. In this patient, the melanoma had already metastasized to the liver.

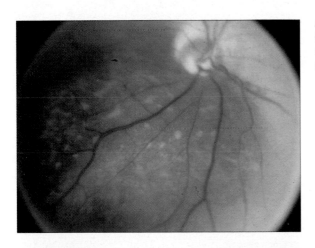

4.19 Circumpapillary malignant melanoma of the choroid with orange lipofuscin pigmentary changes on its surface indicative of the degenerative change in the retinal pigment epithelium.

4.20 Large, elevated solid detachment of the retina with grey colour due to the underlying malignant melanoma of the choroid.

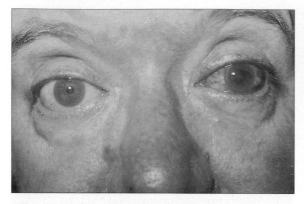

4.21 A 55-year-old white male with acute glaucoma and cataract, which belies underlying malignant melanoma of the choroid.

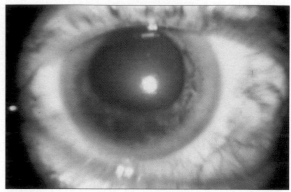

4.22 A high-power photograph of the eye in 4.21 showing the cataract in a compromised angle with a steamy cornea.

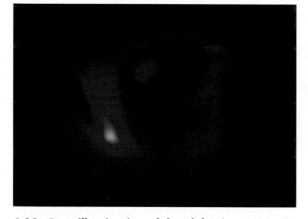

4.23 Retroillumination of the globe demonstrates the inferior pigmentary change of ciliary body melanoma in the patient in **4.21**.

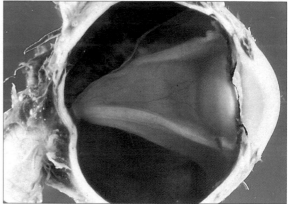

4.24 Gross specimen shows the ciliary body melanoma, which has extended into the choroid and completely detached the retina, pushing the lens and anterior segment structures forward causing the secondary glaucoma and compromise.

4.25 A 51-year-old white female with malignant melanoma (undetected) on back, which has metastatized to the iris and ciliary body, causing uveitis and secondary glaucoma.

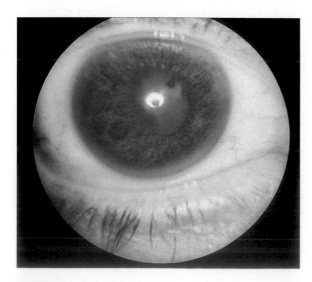

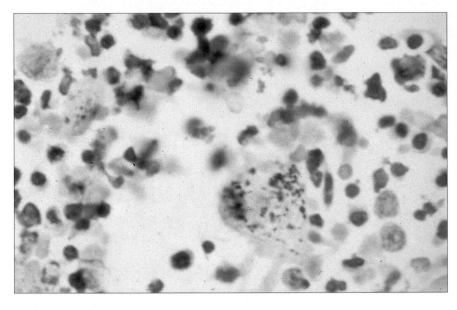

4.26 Histological specimen of aqueous paracentesis of the patient in **4.25** demonstrating obvious and profuse malignant melanoma cells.

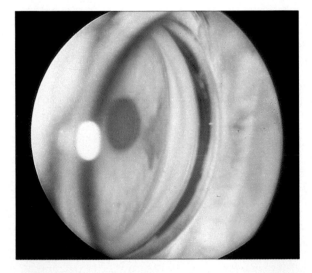

4.27 A 51-year-old white male with malignant melanoma of the iris.

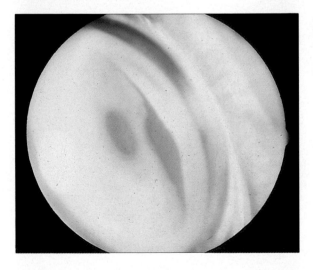

4.28 A 78-year-old white female with ciliary body malignant melanoma, which metastasized contiguously to the iris, giving the false impression of an iris melanoma, which might not otherwise have a serious consequence.

5. Phakomatoses

The phakomatoses: ataxia–telangiectasia, Sturge–Weber syndrome, neurofibromatosis, tuberous sclerosis, von Hippel–Lindau disease, Wyburn–Mason disease

Definition
- Hereditary hamartomatous vascular conditions involving the eye, but also disseminated to the skin and central nervous system, and with profound systemic manifestations. All are autosomal dominant except ataxia–telangiectasia (Louis–Bar syndrome), which is autosomal recessive

Presentation
- Decreased vision due to underlying vascular condition
- Sturge–Weber syndrome: often with glaucoma

Investigation
- Family history
- Intravenous fluorescein angiography for choroidal haemangioma in Sturge–Weber syndrome
- Skull radiograph or scans for central nervous system tumours: cerebellar haemangioblastoma; phaeochromocytoma in von Hippel–Lindau disease; cerebral calcifications/tumours in neurofibromatosis and tuberous sclerosis; optic nerve glioma in neurofibromatosis

Therapy
- Directed at vascular abnormality

Complications
- Depend upon vascular abnormality
- Glaucoma prominent in Sturge–Weber syndrome
- Seizures, cerebrovascular accidents
- Respiratory infections/bronchiectasis and neuropathology in ataxia–telangiectasia

Prognosis
- Variable

Table 5.1 The phakomatoses: ataxia–telangiectasia, Sturge–Weber syndrome, neurofibromatosis, tuberous sclerosis, von Hippel–Lindau disease, Wyburn–Mason disease.

The phakomatoses (**Table 5.1**) derive their name from the Greek for 'mother-spot,' or birthmark. It is used to describe a group of congenital ectodermal dysplasias, typically hamartomas, which occur in the nervous system, skin, eyes and other organs. Six syndromes are currently recognized:
- Neurofibromatosis (von Recklinghausen's disease).
- Tuberous sclerosis (Bourneville's disease).
- Cerebello-retinal haemangioblastomatosis (von Hippel–Lindau disease).
- Encephalotrigeminal angiomatosis (Sturge–Weber syndrome).
- Ataxia–telangiectasia (Louis–Bar syndrome).
- Wyburn–Mason syndrome.

NEUROFIBROMATOSIS

Neurofibromatosis (**5.1 and 5.2**) is a developmental defect of the neuroectoderm (neural crest origin) and is transmitted as an autosomal dominant trait. Pigmented skin lesions called café au lait spots, and multiple neural fibromas occur in association with widespread tumours and other systemic manifestations. This is the classical 'elephant man' disease of legendary Londoner John Merrick.

Neurofibromatosis occurs in 1 in 3000 live births and recent research studies have linked a gene marker to chromosome 17. This finding is expected to aid prenatal and postnatal diagnosis of this disorder.

Almost all structures of the eye may be affected by neurofibromatosis. The cornea may show exposure

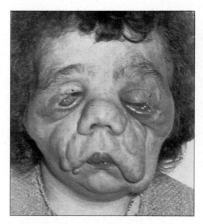

5.1 Profound facial distortion in a young woman with facial neurofibromatosis. Note the tremendous structural malpositioning of the lids and orbital tissue in relationship to the eye.

from lagophthalmos or facial nerve damage, and corneal anaesthesia due to trigeminal nerve damage. Both may be caused by acoustic neuroma.

Thickening of corneal nerves is visible by slit lamp biomicroscopy. The conjunctiva may demonstrate plexiform neuromas and the iris may demonstrate neurofibromas.

Astrocytomas or mulberry lesions may be noted in the retina. The optic nerve is known to demonstrate gliomas, meningiomas, optic atrophy, papilloedema, and myelination of the optic nerve. In addition, proptosis may result from orbital engorgement and erosion of the orbital fissures by meningioma, which may transmit pulsations from the internal carotid artery.

Ptosis may be a consequence of plexiform neuroma of the eyelid; café au lait spots may be noted around the eyelids.

The demonstration of six or more café au lait spots measuring over 1.5 cm is diagnostic for neurofibromatosis in the presence of any of the other designated criteria for the disease.

Glaucoma may also occur due to infiltration of the angle by neurofibroma obstructing aqueous outflow channels. Usually, patients with congenital glaucoma and neurofibromatosis have plexiform neuromas of the ipsilateral eyelid. It has been noted in the literature that 25% of patients with optic glioma have neurofibromatosis, and among these, 15% have tumours of the anterior visual pathways.

Treatment of this disease includes surgery for neurofibromas of the eyelid and orbit, and medical and surgical therapy for glaucoma.

The glaucoma is usually congenital and may occur before other neurological or cutaneous signs of neurofibromatosis.

TUBEROUS SCLEROSIS

Tuberous sclerosis (**5.3–5.8**) is characterized by the clinical triad of adenoma sebaceum, astrocytic haematoma of the retina, and epilepsy. Its classical description was characterized by the acronym EPILOIA,

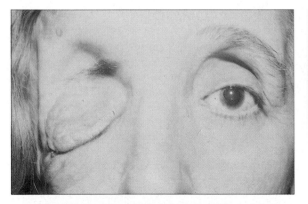

5.2 Plexiform neuroma of the eyelid in a patient with neurofibromatosis. On palpation, this lesion feels rubbery, much like a collection of 'worms' under the surface epidermis.

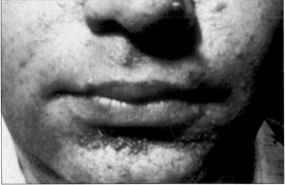

5.3 A patient with adenoma sebaceum over the malar areas and the particularly prominent lesions under the labial folds inferiorly in the chin recess show that these angiofibromas are large elevated nodules and not the abscesses of acne.

5.4 Subungual fibromas in the nail beds of the foot of this 20-year-old patient with tuberous sclerosis.

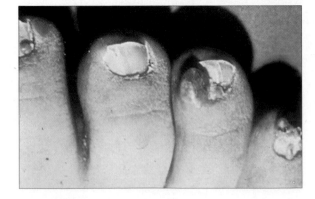

which included the epilepsy, low intelligence and adenoma sebaceum. The original descriptions of this disease were based on institutionalized patients, but it is now known that many patients are not mentally retarded.

Tuberous sclerosis is a dominantly inherited condition with a high rate of new mutation. Patients have hamartomatous lesions in the brain, heart, kidneys, and epididymis, as well as the eyes.

The most characteristic ocular finding is an astrocytic hamartoma of the retina, which is found in 50–80% of examined patients. Histologically, retinal hamartomas consist of astrocytes with long processes and small oval nuclei. They initially arise from retinal ganglion cells, but later involve all layers of the retina.

Adenoma sebaceum is a misnomer and the actual skin manifestations are angiofibromas, which are most frequently found on the face of patients and may be misdiagnosed as acne. The use of a Wood's lamp in a darkened room is helpful in locating these lesions in the skin. Facial angiofibromas are usually present in up to 50% of patients and may be first noted when the patient is 3–5 years of age. They are

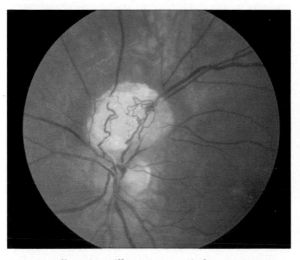

5.5 Small peripapillary astrocytic hamartoma in a patient with tuberous sclerosis.

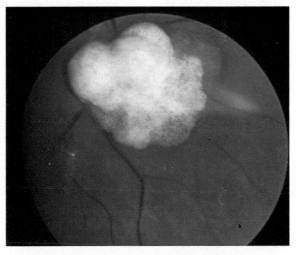

5.6 Large astrocytic hamartoma covering the optic nerve head in a pedunculated fashion. If this patient were much younger, this lesion could easily be confused with a retinoblastoma or a regressing retinoblastoma.

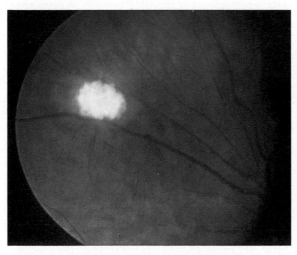

5.7 Very peripheral small focal astrocytic hamartoma in a patient with minimal signs and symptoms of tuberous sclerosis.

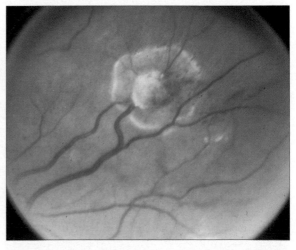

5.8 A small peripheral 'ivory' glistening surface to an astrocytic hamartoma temporal to the macula in a patient with tuberous sclerosis.

usually red, elevated, rubbery nodules, and are typically noted in the nasolabial folds on the chin and over the malar areas.

Fibrous plaques or Shagreen's patches are confluent areas of skin tumour of waxy, yellowish-brown, or flesh-coloured appearance seen elsewhere, and may be found on the forehead, back, or legs. Ungual fibromas may be noted in the fingernails or toenails.

The clinican should also examine teeth for pitted enamel, and while this is rare in the average population, 70% of patients with typical tuberous sclerosis are found to have it.

Hamartomas occur in the kidney, heart and epididymis, and may be angiomyolipomas as well as cysts, which can be found in one or both kidneys of most patients. These can lead to haematuria, uraemia and renal failure, and rarely hypertension.

VON HIPPEL–LINDAU DISEASE

Von Hippel–Lindau disease (**5.9–5.16**) is the association of angioblastic tumours of the retina and haemangioblastomas of the cerebellum and viscera.

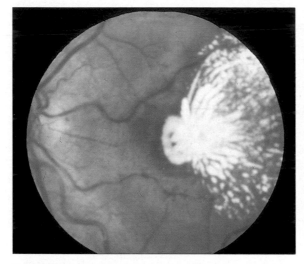

5.9 A 7-year-old white male with von Hippel–Lindau disease demonstrating a macular star with exudation in the nerve fibre layer of the macula in the left eye.

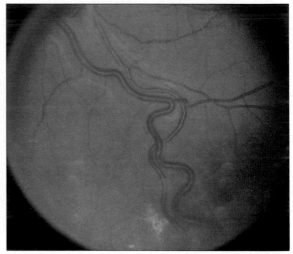

5.10 Same eye of the patient, following feeder vessels, which are large and tortuous inferotemporally from the optic nerve.

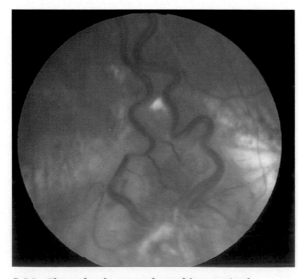

5.11 These feeder vessels end in a retinal angioma as noted in this clinical photograph.

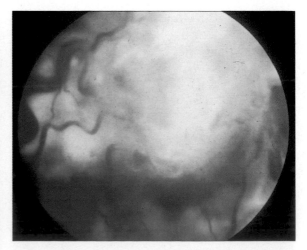

5.12 Different patient showing large peripheral dome-shaped retinal angioma with two large feeder vessels, one on either side, showing marked tumour formation in a patient with von Hippel–Lindau's disease.

Involvement of the kidney may lead to polycythaemia, possibly as a result of an increased production of erythropoietin. The condition is transmitted as an autosomal dominant, but may arise spontaneously. It is considered to be a developmental dysgenesis of both neuroectoderm and mesoderm.

Five neoplastic lesions may produce morbidity and even death in these patients:

- Cerebellar angioma.
- Medullary angioma.
- Spinal haemangioblastoma.
- Renal cell carcinoma.
- Phaeochromocytoma.

In contrast, there are commonly more cysts than angiomatous tumours of several visceral organs and these may be asymptomatic.

Cerebellar haemangioblastoma is the commonest central nervous system manifestation of the disease and is reported in 35–75% in families. The tumour is usually asymptomatic until the second to fourth decade of life, and while it is usually a resectable lesion, it is also the most common cause of death.

Angiomatosis of the retina is found in the majority of these patients. Tumours are often mid-peripheral or peripheral in location and may be diagnosed as a secondary consequence of macular oedema and even 'star' formation with large feeder vessels lead-

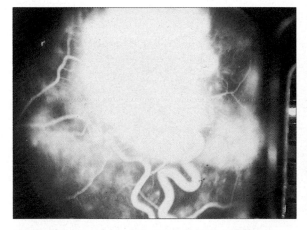

5.13 Fluorescein angiogram showing diffuse staining and uptake of fluorescein. Note the demarcation between the afferent and the efferent feeder vessels inferiorly in this large peripheral retinal angioma.

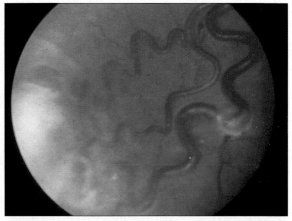

5.14 A different patient with a retinal angioma peripherally. Note that there is one large afferent feeder vessel extending to it and two efferent feeding vessels extending from it.

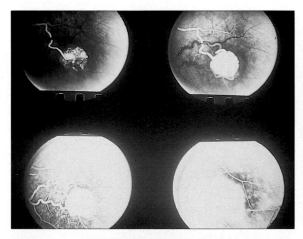

5.15 A composite slide of fluorescein angiogram of a von Hippel–Lindau's peripheral retinal angioma, which is well circumscribed. Note the early filling, which outlines its morphology in the late filling, which stains beyond it.

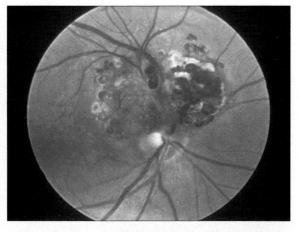

5.16 An atypical retinal angioma peripherally in a 30-year-old white male with von Hippel–Lindau's disease.

ing out to the tumours through surrounding exudative retinal detachment.

Treatment includes photocoagulation, which necessitates treatment to the feeder vessels first, and is then later applied directly to the surface of the angioma. Cryotherapy, and occasionally diathermy, which may successfully obliterate the angioma primarily, treats the macular oedema secondarily.

ENCEPHALOTRIGEMINAL ANGIOMATOSIS (STURGE–WEBER SYNDROME)

Encephalotrigeminal angiomatosis, or Sturge–Weber syndrome (**5.17–5.27**), is a nonfamilial disorder of capillary or cavernous haemangiomas occurring in the skin of the face in the dermatomes supplied by the trigeminal nerve. Intracranial haemangiomas in the leptomeninges are associated with calcifications of the underlying cerebral cortex, which give rise to seizure disorders and perhaps mental retardation.

The ocular manifestations of this disease include the dermatome cavernous haemangiomas or capillary haemangiomas (naevus flammeus) around the eyes and causing secondary glaucoma, as well as accompanying conjunctival, episcleral, iris, and choroidal involvement. Secondary cataract formation and optic atrophy may also occur.

A pathognomonic feature of the Sturge–Weber syndrome is an angioma of the pia and the arachnoid matter. The vascular circulation in the underlying

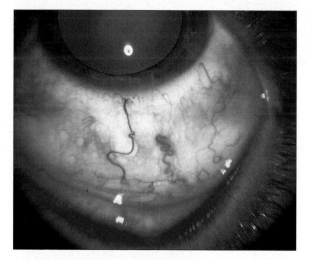

5.17 Very subtle epibulbar telangiectasis in a patient with a choroidal haemangioma and Sturge–Weber syndrome.

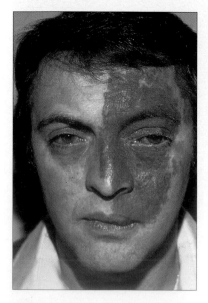

5.18 Giant facial naevus in a patient with Sturge–Weber syndrome. Note how the demarcations of this naevus flammeus exquisitely follow the facial dermatomes.

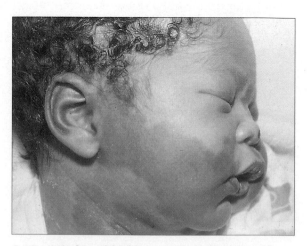

5.19 A 2-day-old African–American male with Sturge–Weber syndrome demonstrating a large and diffuse facial haemangioma, choroidal haemangioma, and glaucoma.

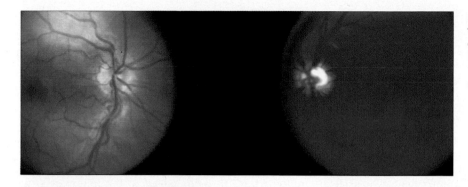

5.20 Compare two fundi of young male with choroidal beet-coloured hemangioma, glaucoma and "cupped" optic disk in left retina.

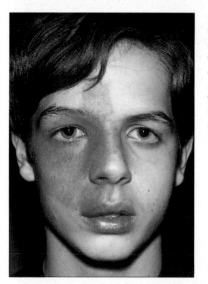

5.21 A youngster demonstrating the exquisitely demarcated naevus flammeus following the dermatome.

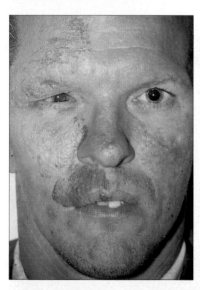

5.22 Large elevated choroidal haemangioma inferiorly in a 15-year-old patient with Sturge–Weber syndrome.

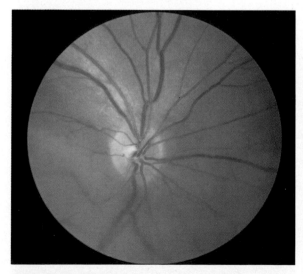

5.23 Very peripheral and very elevated choroidal haemangioma in the same patient as in 5.22.

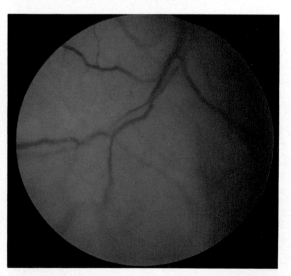

5.24 Same eye in the 15-year-old patient shown in 5.22 with choroidal haemangioma inferiorly showing an area superiorly that probably represents a spontaneously resorbed and now somewhat calcified subretinal area corresponding to a previous haemangioma.

cerebral cortex may be abnormal as a consequence. Either focal or generalized seizures are noted in 80% of patients. Intracranial calcifications are therefore common in the majority of these patients and may be detected from the first or second decade of life.

Approximately 30% of patients with Sturge–Weber syndrome are noted to develop glaucoma. Of these, 60% present before the age of two years with buphthalmos, and the remaining 40% do not develop glaucoma until late childhood or young adulthood. Most commonly this is unilateral. The intraocular pressure is often elevated in the patients whose facial naevus flammeus involves the eyelid or conjunctiva. While the cause of the glaucoma remains enigmatic, it is thought to be due to an outflow obstruction by chamber angle malformation or occlusion of the angle with anterior synechiae.

Choroidal haemangioma also occurs and is typically situated temporal to the optic disc with its greatest height in the macular region. However, initial ophthalmoscopic appearance may be misleading since the tumour may be so extensive that the deep red colour of this choroidal haemangioma may not be noticed until it is compared to the fellow eye. In

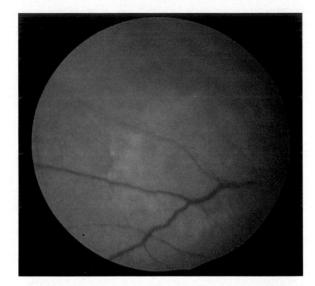

5.25 Subtle area of telangiectasis on episclera and sclera of patient with chronic glaucoma and choroidal haemangioma with Sturge–Weber syndrome.

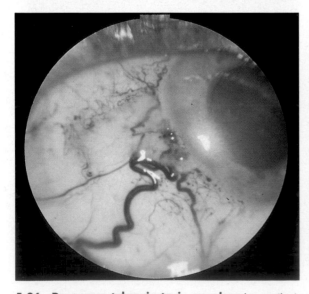

5.26 Racemose telangiectasis on sclera in a patient with Sturge–Weber syndrome.

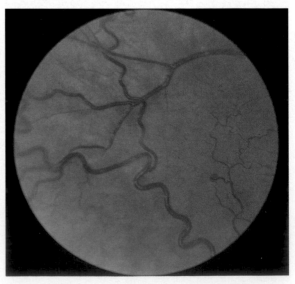

5.27 Capillary haemangioma of the optic nerve head demonstrating a mulberry surface appearance with some sclerosis and calcification.

particular, asymmetry of the optic nerve heads between the two eyes should be looked for if a choroidal haemangioma has a subtle appearance. Rarely, calcification may occur in an angiomatosis choroid, and some patients who present at a young age with an idiopathic subretinal calcification syndrome are thought to have degenerated choroidal angiomas, an incomplete form of Sturge–Weber syndrome. Other ocular abnormalities noted in this disorder are retinal vessel tortuosity, retinitis pigmentosa, neuroblastoma of the retina, bilateral lens subluxation, and anisocoria coloboma of the iris and optic nerve head.

ATAXIA–TELANGIECTASIA (LOUIS–BAR SYNDROME)

Ataxia–telangiectasia or the Louis–Bar syndrome is an autosomal recessive disorder that involves the skin, central nervous system, haematopoietic and lymphoreticular system, as well as the eye. It is characterized by progressive cerebellar ataxia, telangiectatic lesions of the lid and conjunctiva, and a generalized immunological incompetence with a deficiency of IgA and delayed hypersensitivity. Recurrent infections, especially pulmonary infections, may result in early death. It has been noted that the disorder appears to result from failure of the thymus to develop, and there is also a incomplete absence of IgE and IgG and a deficiency of T cell function. Patients have an increased risk of developing leukaemia, malignant lymphoma, and other systemic malignancies.

Patients with ataxia–telangiectasia show a variety of abnormalities of ocular motility in addition to the almost universal finding of conjunctival telangiecta-sia. They may be unable to initiate voluntary saccades and abnormalities in the fast phase of vestibular nystagmus. Pursuit movements are impaired and there may even be a late and total ophthalmoplegia.

The neuropathology of ataxia–telangiectasia consists of atrophy of the cerebellar cortex, particularly with an absence of Purkinje and granular cells. This is associated with the reduction of neurotransmitters including glutamate, taurine, and γ-aminobutyric acid. The prognosis for quality and length of life is poor.

WYBURN–MASON SYNDROME

Wyburn–Mason syndrome, which is also called Bonet–Dechaume–Blanc (**5.28–5.30**) is a combination of retinal and systemic arteriovenous malformations (AVMs). These malformations consist of direct communication between the arterial and venous circulation and involve predominantly the central nervous system, the ocular adnexa, and the oropharynx. AVMs are the most common form of intracranial vascular hamartoma and the majority are found in and associated with the middle cerebral artery, but they may involve various sites of the visual pathways resulting in papilloedema, optic atrophy, or hemianopia. The other manifestations of central nervous system AVMs include headaches, seizures, mental retardation, cranial nerve palsy, and hemiparesis. They may be associated with intracerebral or subarachnoid haemorrhage and therefore have a potentially lethal prognosis. Epistaxis with neural haemorrhage, especially during dental procedures, may be the presenting sign of nasopharyngeal AVMs.

AVMs involving the orbit and eyelids produce ptosis, proptosis, dilated conjunctival vessels and

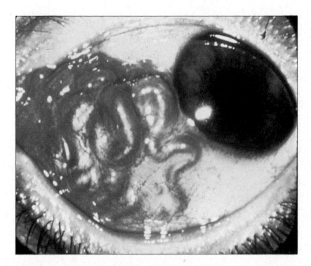

5.28 Wyburn–Mason arteriovenous malformation in the retina in a patient who also had a submandibular malformation, which was noted on tooth extraction at the dentist to cause profuse bleeding and led to a transfusion in hospital.

bruits. Retinal AVMs are congenital and stable, and are usually unilateral vascular malformations that have a predilection for the posterior pole and superotemporal quadrant. Although most retinal AVMs are stable, several complications have been reported including intraretinal macular haemorrhage, central retinal vein occlusion, branch retinal vein occlusion, avascular glaucoma and vitreous haemorrhage. Some retinal AVMs may undergo spontaneous regression following retinal vein occlusion. Venous occlusive disease is related to the 'arterialization' of the venous system.

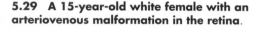

5.29 A 15-year-old white female with an arteriovenous malformation in the retina.

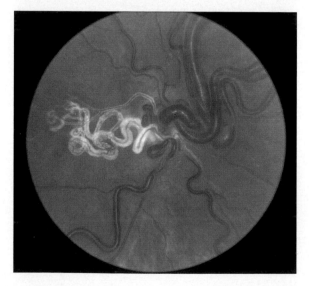

5.30 A more peripheral area of tortuous and abnormal blood vessels distal to the arteriovenous malformation of the patient in **5.29**.

6. Metabolic Disorders

RETINITIS PIGMENTOSA

Retinitis pigmentosa is a misnomer. The disease represents a primary degeneration of the retina, especially the photoreceptors, and may be inherited in all genetic patterns. It presents as an independent ophthalmological disorder leading to progressive loss of peripheral vision and night blindness, and may include the ocular features of cataract, myopia, optic atrophy, and attenuation of the retinal vessels. It may be part of a systemic disorder and numerous syndromes have been described, in many of which the underlying metabolic disorder has yet to be elucidated. The most common are:

- Laurence–Moon–Biedl syndrome, which includes retinitis pigmentosa with obesity, mental retardation, polydactyly and hypogonadism.
- Bassen–Kornzweig syndrome (abetalipoproteinemia) is retinitis pigmentosa with acanthosis of the red blood cells, malabsorption of fat, and a spinocerebellar ataxia.
- Refsum's disease (phytanic acid storage disease), which is retinitis pigmentosa with cerebellar ataxia and progressive peripheral polyneuritis.
- Usher's syndrome, an autosomal recessive condition, which is retinitis pigmentosa with deafness. The deafness is a sensorineural deafness that is usually present from birth or noted shortly thereafter.

While other forms of retinitis pigmentosa have been noted, they all share in common a scattered area of pigmentary disturbance in the ocular fundus with a pale optic nerve and attenuation of the retinal vasculature. 'Bone corpuscle' configuration is a characteristic sign of the retinal pigmentary degeneration, and the abnormal pigment usually overlies the retinal vessels (**6.1–6.4**). This disease is a degeneration of the retina, and not an inflammatory condition as its name implies.

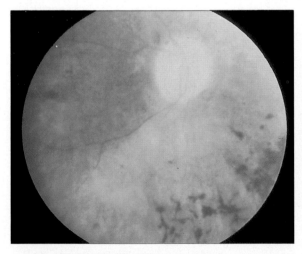

6.1   Typical fundal findings of retinitis pigmentosa, including a pale disc, attenuation of the retinal vasculature and the darkly pigmented bone spicules disseminated through the retina.

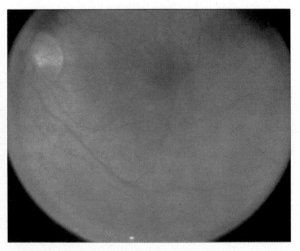

6.2   More marked attenuation of retinal vasculature, but with less prominent distribution of bone spicules through the retina of a patient with retinitis pigmentosa.

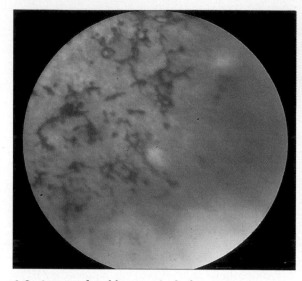

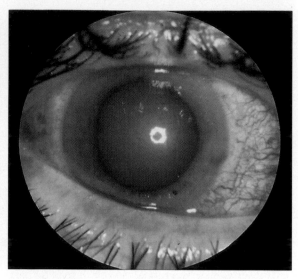

6.3 Intense focal bone spicule formation in one quadrant of the eye in a patient with retinitis pigmentosa.

6.4 A 40-year-old white male with dense cataract formation in retinitis pigmentosa.

INHERITED METABOLIC DISORDERS WITH OPHTHALMOLOGICAL FEATURES

Many inherited metabolic disorders are associated with ophthalmological signs and symptoms. Some are prominently known in ophthalmology such as:

- Wilson's disease in which Kayser–Fleischer rings, a bluish-green deposition in Bowman's membrane of the cornea, are prominent. Sunflower cataract is also pathognomonic of Wilson's disease, due to an inability of the liver to metabolize copper.
- Abnormal amino acid metabolism is represented by homocystinuria and albinism, while abnormal carbohydrate metabolism represented by galactosaemia, may present as a reversible cataract in infants.
- Disorders of lipid and lipoprotein metabolism (6.5–6.7) are among those most frequently presenting with ocular abnormalities and represent the hyperlipidaemia syndromes.

Retinitis pigmentosa may represent some inborn error of metabolism since it is neither an inflammation of the retina nor is the visual loss related to pigment deposition.

Ectopia lentis may be noted in homocystinuria, galactosaemia, Marfan's syndrome.

Lipaemia retinalis, a striking fundal picture of white–yellow vessels coloured by the lipid burden in the vascular system, occurs when the triglyceride level exceeds 2000 mg/ml.

THE GANGLIOSIDOSES

The gangliosidoses, which include Tay–Sachs disease and Sandhoff's disease, are represented as inherited conditions whose basic defect is the insufficient activity of the lysosomal enzyme, which results in the accumulation of abnormal substances in various tissues. While this produces the ocular sign of a 'cherry red spot' in an infant as a consequence of perimacular glycolipid deposition in the retinal ganglion cells, optic atrophy and pigmentary retinal degeneration may be the more obvious and harmful ocular complications secondary to the spinocerebellar dysfunction and upper and lower motor neuron involvement of this disease, which often leads to death from central nervous system involvement.

Gaucher's disease and other inherited disorders of glycolipid metabolism involve serious bone disease and hepatosplenomegaly, and are due to excessive accumulation of glucocerebroside in the liver and bone marrow. White deposits, which probably represent lipid-laden macrophages, have been described in the corneal epithelium. Vitreous opacities and cells have been reported, with the cherry red spot similar to that seen in Tay–Sachs disease, perimacular pigmentary changes, and characteristic white spots in the retina.

MUCOPOLYSACCHARIDOSES

The mucopolysaccharide storage diseases, which result from a deficiency of enzymes involving the

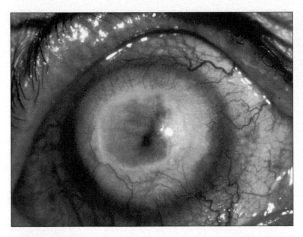

6.5   Lipoidal corneal dystrophy in the peripheral cornea.

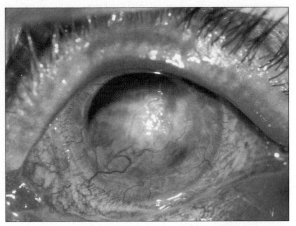

6.6   Central lipoid deposits in the lipoidal dystrophy.

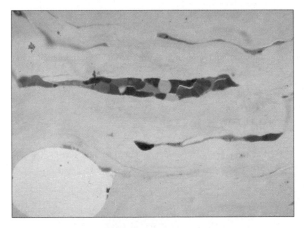

6.7   Histological demonstration of lipoidal deposits in the cornea.

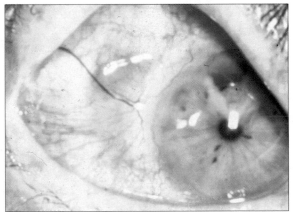

6.8   Scleral ectasia underlying acute scleritis and corneal melting syndrome secondary to gout.

degradation of glycosaminoglycans, also result in connective tissue disease involvement. They have a varying degree of severity and overlap and cause skeletal abnormalities, typical facial structural abnormalities, hepatosplenomegaly, cardiac disease, mental deficiency, deafness, and of course, ocular manifestations. The variability in the clinical features is due to tissue specific differences and where the mucopolysaccharides are accumulated. All cause corneal clouding, some pigmentary retinal dystrophies, and optic atrophy.

Hurler's syndrome usually becomes manifest by 2–3 years of age with dwarfism and the typical facial features. Corneal clouding is diffuse and the fundal picture reveals a retinitis pigmentosa-like picture indistinguishable from the other pigmentary dystrophies. There is narrowing of the retinal vasculature and optic atrophy is seen. Scheie's syndrome may involve a similar enzyme defect to that of Hurler's

syndrome and even Hunter's syndrome, and is an X-linked recessive disorder that appears in early infancy. It later manifests with its typical facial appearance, stiff joints, deafness, short stature, heart disease, hepatosplenomegaly, and nodular skin lesions. While corneal clouding may not be common in Hunter's syndrome, deposits of acid mucopolysaccharide may be found histologically in clinically clear corneas.

Sanfilippo's, Morquio's and Maroteaux–Lamy syndromes are the other recognized mucopolysaccharide storage defects with ocular signs and symptoms. No retinal dystrophy has been noted in Morquio's syndrome, while in Sanfilippo's syndrome, pigmentary retinal degeneration similar to retinitis pigmentosa with vascular narrowing and optic atrophy is typical. Maroteaux–Lamy syndrome causes hydrocephalus secondary to meningeal involvement and may lead to death in the early years of life.

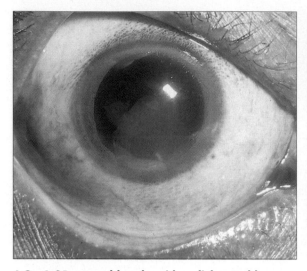

6.9 A 21-year-old male with a dislocated lens, a feature of Marfan's syndrome.

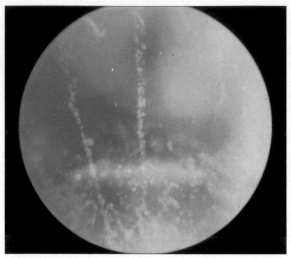

6.10 A 'starry night' vitreous indicative of **asteroid hyalitis**.

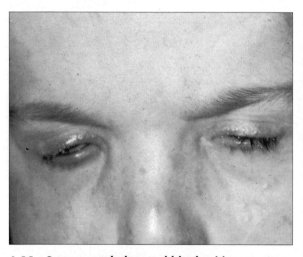

6.11 Severe staphylococcal blepharitis in a patient with immunodeficiency disorder.

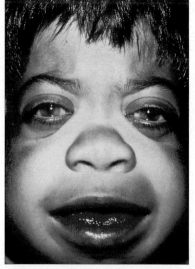

6.12 Classical facies of Hurler's syndrome.

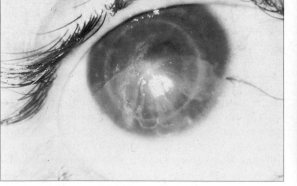

6.13 Acute corneal changes in Reilly–Day syndrome.

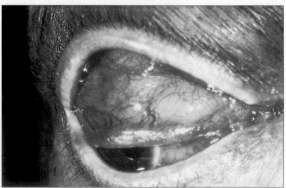

6.14 Proptosis secondary to amyloid deposition in the orbit.

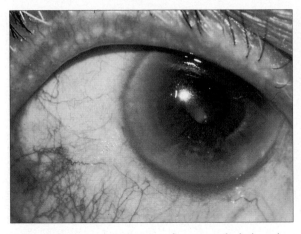

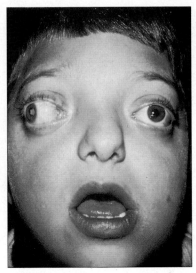

6.15 Bitot's spots. Glistening, foamy paralimbal patches of cornified epithelium suggestive of generalized malnutrition and vitamin A deficiency in particular.

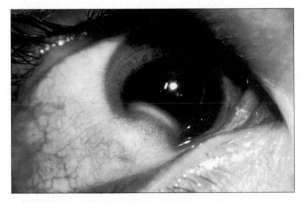

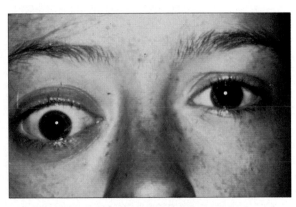

6.17 Limbal dermoid in a patient with Goldenhar's syndrome.

6.18 Proptosis with infratemporal displacement of globe and corneal exposure in a young boy with fibrous dysplasia.

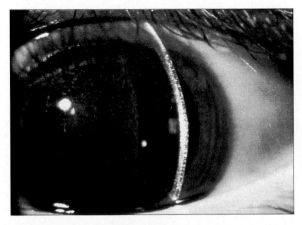

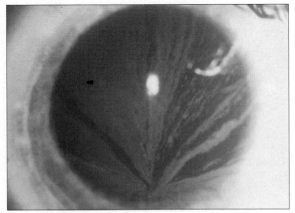

6.19 Cystinosis of the cornea in a 9-year-old male.

6.20 A 29-year-old white female with Fabry's disease and typical corneal changes. (Courtesy of R.L. Abbott, MD.)

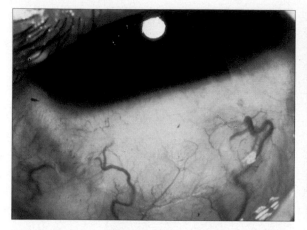

6.21 Epibulbar telangiectasis and inflammation in a child with Hand–Schüller–Christian disease.

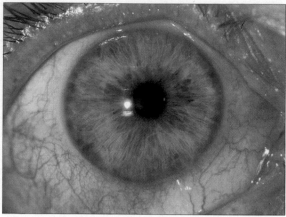

6.22 Acute dry eye syndrome with Rose Bengal staining in a patient with connective tissue disease.

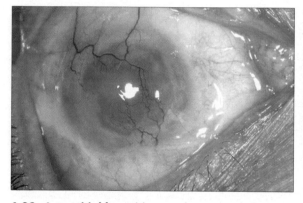

6.23 Interstitial keratitis secondary to metabolic dysfunction.

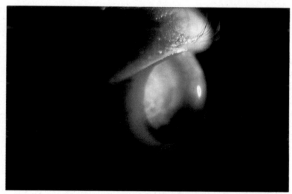

6.24 A patient with keratoconus and cataract in Down's syndrome.

6.25 Uric acid deposits in the cornea in a patient with gout.

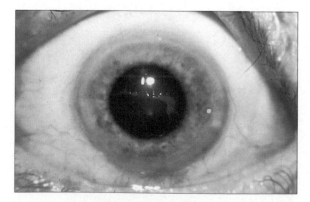

7.
Infections and Infestations of the Eye and Adnexa

Types of organism causing eye infections

Viruses	Herpes viruses
	    Herpes simplex
	    Herpes zoster
	    CMV (cytomegalovirus)
	    Epstein–Barr virus
	Human immunodeficiency virus (HIV)
	Influenza
	Measles
	Molluscum contagiosum
	Mumps
	Rubella
	Subacute sclerosing panencephalitis
	Varicella
		Chlamydia
		
		Myobacteria
		
		Fungal
			Trachoma
			'Venereal' conjunctivitis
			
			Tubercolosis
			Leprosy
			
			Candida albicans
			Aspergillosis
			Histoplasmosis
			Metastatic
			Fungal
			Ophthalmitis
			(Drug abuse, AIDS)

Bacteria	Staphylococci Streptococci *Pneumocytosis carinii* Botulism Brucellosis Diphtheria Tularaemia Metastatic bacterial Ophthalmitis	**Spirochaetes** **Parasites**	Lyme disease Leptospirosis Relapsing fever Syphilis Toxoplasmosis *Toxocara canis* Trypanosomiasis Malaria Leishmaniasis Amoebiasis
Helminths	Cysticercosis Hydatid disease Loa loa Onchocerciasis Schistosomiasis	**Rickettsiae**	Rocky Mountain spotted fever Q fever

Table 7.1   Types of organism causing eye infections.

The eye may be involved in almost any type of systemic infection, inflammation or infestation (**Table 7.1**). The noninfectious inflammations of unknown aetiology will be discussed in another chapter, but the eye may manifest primary infections in the ocular tissue due to viruses, bacteria, chlamydia, helminthic disease, mycobacteria, fungi, protozoans, rickettsiae, and spirochaetes. It may also be a distant focus for systemic infection from all of these infectious agents.

The viral infections of the herpetic family have caused increasing morbidity and interest over the years. They are also more frequent now. Herpes simplex and zoster are always common in serious diseases of the cornea, but cytomegalovirus (CMV) has become an increasingly frequent herpes infection because of its association with the acquired immunodeficiency syndrome (AIDS) pandemic.

VIRAL INFECTIONS

HERPES VIRUS

The herpes virus family consisting of DNA viruses is attracting increasing attention from clinicians and researchers because of its high prevalence in the population both as a venereal infection and otherwise.

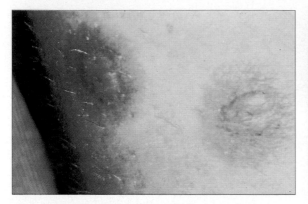

7.1   Epidermal vesicle formation, herpes simplex disease.

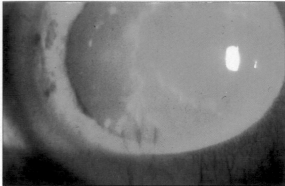

7.2   More ropy, more extensive fluorescein-stained dendrites, herpes simplex disease.

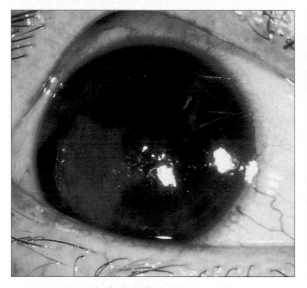

7.3   Large epithelial defect filled in with fluorescein dye in a patient with herpes simplex disease.

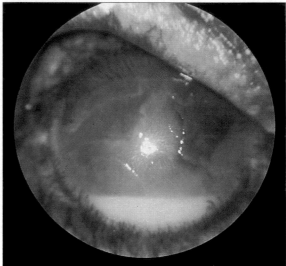

7.4   Geographical ulcer of epithelium with hypopyon formation in very profound herpes simplex virus infection.

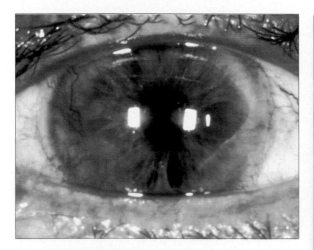

7.5   Stromal scarring in a patient with herpes simplex infection.

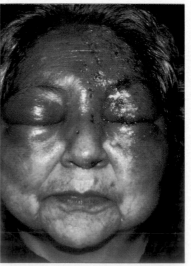

7.6   A 68-year-old woman with lymphoma who manifested herpes zoster ophthalmicus over the entire maxillary distribution of that facial dermatome.

The herpes family includes:
- Herpes simplex virus (HSV), sometimes referred to as herpes hominis.
- Herpes zoster virus.
- CMV.
- Epstein–Barr virus.

All cause ocular inflammation, but have varying manifestations of disease.

Herpes simplex

Herpes simplex (**7.1–7.5, Table 7.2**) usually causes keratitis, both with stromal and disciform lesions, which may be accompanied by an anterior segment inflammation with chronic precipitates. This may sometimes initiate a recurring iridocyclitis, which may occur in the absence of active keratitis. Acute or chronic glaucoma may complicate the iridocyclitis.

Herpes simplex virus has been isolated from the aqueous humour and has been noted by electron microscopy in the iris and stroma. Antibody titres to the herpes viruses are usually of little diagnostic significance because of its ubiquitous nature. Routine studies done in both infants and adults show that there is over 90% positivity in patients who have no known herpes infection. Herpes simplex may rarely cause a retinal inflammation in the newborn or in immunodepressed patients who are debilitated.

Herpes zoster

Herpes zoster ophthalmicus (**7.6–7.9, Table 7.2**) may often be accompanied by iridocyclitis and vitritis. There may be hyphaema, hypopyon, and vitreous involvement in severe cases; optic nerve infection may also occur. The iridocyclitis may be profound, but the virus has only rarely been recovered from the aqueous in patients with this infection.

Herpes virus 1: herpes 1 simplex, herpes 2 genital, herpes zoster

Definition
- Iritis
- Iridocyclitis
- Keratouveitis chronology, either acute or chronic
- Granulomatous

Investigation
- Diagnosis based on previous history of herpetic corneal disease
- Test for corneal sensation
- Skin lesion in zoster or look for previous keratitis

Therapy
- Topical antivirals
- Systemic acyclovir
- Topical steroids may be necessary with antiviral coverage
- Glaucoma therapy, if necessary

Complications
- Glaucoma
- Cataract
- Corneal scarring and vascularization

Prognosis
- Fair in absence of glaucoma or scarring
- Poor if glaucoma scarring or frequent recurrences and poor response to treatment
- May be extremely sensitive to steroid treatment and, therefore, steroid reduction

Table 7.2 Herpes virus 1: herpes 1 simplex, herpes 2 genital, herpes zoster.

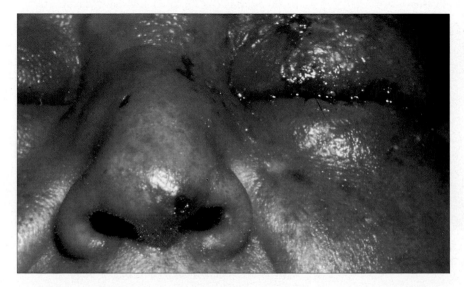

7.7 Close-up showing the nasociliary branch distribution of her herpes zoster infection, which is a clinical sign indicative of ocular involvement.

Often patients with diabetes mellitus or lymphoma are more prone to the infection, but the patient does not need to be immunocompromised.

Herpes zoster virus has a predilection for neural tissue and may cause an intense perineuritis and perivasculitis in and around the optic nerve head.

Herpes virus 2: Epstein–Barr virus

Definition
- Iritis
- Iridocyclitis
- Can be keratitis
- Can be choroiditis
- Acute and chronic

Presentation
- Granulomatous

Investigation
- Titres of anticapsidigms and early antigen demonstration

Therapy
- Acyclovir, prednisolone, topical steroids and mydriatics

Complications
- Synechiae
- Cataract
- Glaucoma
- Cystoid macular oedema
- Possible subretinal neovascular membrane

Prognosis
- Poor if posterior pole is involved

Table 7.3 Herpes virus 2: Epstein–Barr.

Cytomegalovirus inclusion disease

CMV causes a distinctive retinitis in newborns, infants, and immunocompromised adults who are usually undergoing organ transplant surgery or cancer therapy, or who have AIDS. There is an exudative retinitis with occlusive necrotizing vasculitis and retinal hemorrhage, described as 'pizza pie' retinopathy (**7.10 and 7.11, Table 7.4**).

Serological assessment has revealed that a high percentage of the normal population has been exposed to this virus. However, very rarely, some seemingly healthy patients may have the ARN or BARN syndrome (see below) as a possible consequence of CMV inclusion disease (CID) in the retina.

CMV is an opportunist that causes significant ocular disease in infants and small children or in compromised adult hosts. The iridocyclitis that occurs is usually secondary to the necrotizing occlusive vasculitis seen in the retina. There is often a moderate number of cells in the vitreous and vitreous precipitates, which appear on the posterior vitreous face and the internal limiting membrane of the retina. Large areas of confluent retinal necrosis are caused by the neural cell-to-cell transmission of this virus. The retina may take on a grey-brown, totally necrotic appearance. Vessels become sheathed with perivascular accumulations of monoclear inflammatory cell infiltrations.

The typical clinical appearance of CID in an adult who has had either an organ transplantation (kidney or heart) or is otherwise immunosuppressed (i.e. due to cancer chemotherapy) may be enough to substantiate a clinical diagnosis. It is the most common infectious manifestation of ocular AIDS. The disease usually occurs bilaterally, but can be more pronounced in one eye.

CID has increasingly been found to be responsive to zidovudine (AZT), ganciclovir and foscarnet.

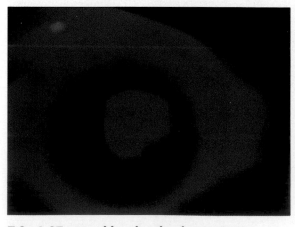

7.8 A 37-year-old male who demonstrates marked iris atrophy from herpes zoster infection.

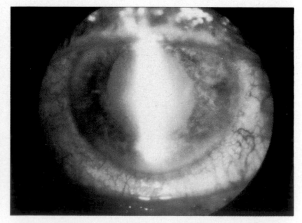

7.9 A 42-year-old white male with extensive depigmentation and atrophy of the iris pigment epithelium from previous herpes zoster infection.

Herpes virus 3: cytomegalovirus inclusion disease

Definition
- Retinitis

Presentation
- Acute
- Granulomatous

Investigation
- Laboratory workup
- Viral studies of urine and serum and titres
- Paediatric consultation
- Complement-fixing antibodies
- Human immunodeficiency virus (HIV) test

Therapy
- DHPGH. Ganciclovir is a new effective, antiviral agent. Recurrences may occur after the drug is stopped or tapered
- Foscarnet. Recent collaborative study demonstrates efficacy to lengthen patient's life
- High doses of systemic steroids and immunosuppressants unless contraindicated

Complications
- Usually a complication of acquired immunodeficiency syndrome (AIDS)
- Drug abuse, organ transplantation, exogenous or endogenous immunosuppression

Prognosis
- Poor, especially in patients with AIDS

Table 7.4   Herpes virus 3: cytomegalovirus inclusion disease.

BILATERAL ACUTE RETINAL NECROSIS (BARN SYNDROME OR ARN SYNDROME)

Acute retinal necrosis (**7.12–7.14, Table 7.5**) is a very severe manifestation of ocular inflammation which occurs in men and women of almost any age. These patients are otherwise healthy and have no systemic prodromal complaints. There is increasing evidence that the syndrome may be related to a CMV or herpes simplex infection. Interestingly, patients who have CMV retinitis in the usual sense are infants or immunoincompetent patients who are compromised by either steroids as part of cancer treatment or organ transplantation or have AIDS.

The onset of the syndrome is abrupt. Vision usually deteriorates rapidly in the first eye and quite significantly in the second eye. Although usually affected some time later, the second eye may remain symptomless for a year or more after the onset of the disease. Only occasionally is one eye alone affected.

The major fundal picture includes severe retinal necrosis with occlusive vasculitis and generalized oedema of the whole retina, with a peripheral whitening spreading to the macular region. As the disease progresses, there is haemorrhage into and in front of the retina and the formation of retinal tears and holes, marked vitreous traction, and often inoperable retinal detachment with consequent phthisis.

Laser photocoagulation to the peripheral necrotic retina may prevent or stall retinal detachment. Most recently, herpes viruses (herpes zoster, 1982; herpes simplex, CMV, Epstein–Barr virus) have been

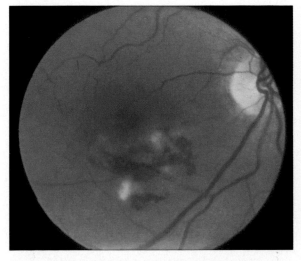

7.10   Cytomegalovirus infection of the retina in a breast cancer patient taking azathioprine.

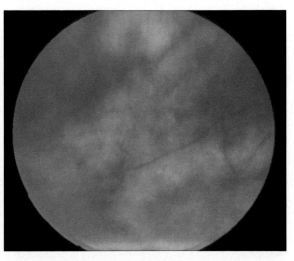

7.11   Peripheral retina demonstrating 'pizza pie' haemorrhagic and necrotic retinopathy of cytomegalovirus infection.

thought to mediate this disease. Treatment with acyclovir is advocated by most authorities. The disease usually progresses rapidly, in a matter of days to weeks. There is an associated mild to moderate anterior inflammation, often with minimal keratic precipitate formation. Usually, the final and catastrophic visual outcome is no light perception in an eye with a necrotic detached retina.

Herpes virus 4: acute retinal necrosis

Definition
- Retinitis
- Vitreoretinitis

Presentation
- Acute
- Granulomatous

Investigation
- Herpes simplex, herpes zoster titres (serum/vitreous)
- Corneal/retinal biopsy (demonstrated virus)

Therapy
- Systemic acyclovir
- ? Intravitreal acyclovir
- Photocoagulation posterior to area of necrosis if visibility allows (to prevent retinal detachment from necrotic thin retina)
- Retinoscopy with broad posterior scleral buckle if retinal detachment develops or if photocoagulation deemed necessary

Complications
- Retinal detachment occurs in more than 75% of patients
- Optic atrophy
- Retinal pucker

Prognosis
- Poor

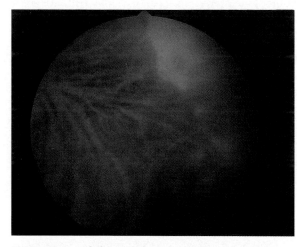

7.12   Very subtle peripheral retinal necrosis in a patient with acute retinal necrosis syndrome.

Table 7.5   Herpes virus 4: acute retinal necrosis.

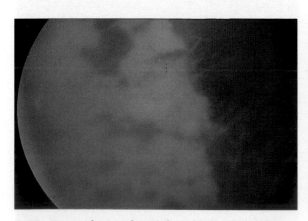

7.13   Very advanced peripheral retinal necrotic change marching toward the posterior pole in patient with acute retinal necrosis syndrome.

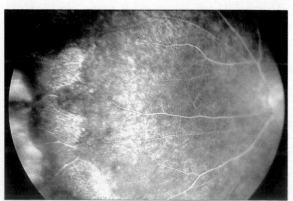

7.14   Fluorescein angiogram of patient in 7.13 demonstrating the edge of the marked retinal necrosis and retinal pigment epithelial change adjacent to it showing more profound fluorescein angiographic abnormalities than in the previous clinical photograph.

ACUTE MULTIFOCAL PLACOID PIGMENT EPITHELIOPATHY

Acute multifocal placoid pigment epitheliopathy (AMPPE, **7.15–7.17, Table 7.6**) is a postdromal viral illness that usually causes an intraocular inflammation limited to retinal pigment epithelium and follows on the heels of an upper respiratory illness, sometimes with headache and erythema nodosum. There is usually an abrupt deterioration of vision in an otherwise symptom-free eye. While the disease is usually bilateral, one eye is often affected before and sometimes more severely than the other. In many instances, it may be difficult to elicit the previous viral symptoms, which have usually occurred several days to several weeks before.

Clinically, grey-white deep retinal lesions are found in the retinal pigment epithelium or in the choriocapillaris and frequently affect the macula. There are paracentral or central scotomas and central vision is reduced.

The degree of visual reduction depends upon the location of the inflammatory lesions. There are usually cells in the vitreous overlying this posterior inflammation and only occasionally with a mild iridocyclitis present. Serous detachment of the retina is rare, but has been reported.

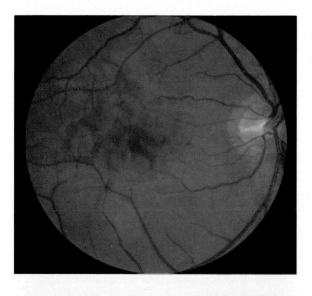

7.15 Acute multifocal placoid pigment epitheliopathy with gross retinal pigment epithelial disturbance changes in the macula. This is thought to be a viral exanthem of the retinal pigment epithelium.

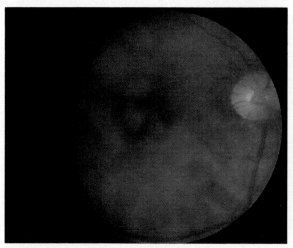

7.16 A 27-year-old patient with acute multifocal placoid pigment epitheliopathy showing marked pigment disturbance in the macula.

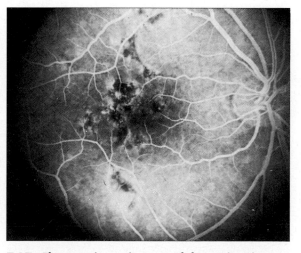

7.17 Fluorescein angiogram of the patient in 7.16 showing how much more profound the fluorescein angiographic changes are than in the clinical photograph.

This inflammatory disorder usually resolves over several weeks, often with scarring and alterations in the appearance of the retinal pigment epithelium and the choriocapillaris. However, the vision frequently returns to normal.

MULTIPLE EVANESCENT WHITE DOT SYNDROME

Multiple evanescent white dot syndrome (MEWDS, **Table 7.7**) is an inflammation of the retinal pigment epithelium (RPE), choriocapillaris, and Bruch's membrane and overlaps into the neurosensory retina. It is an entity with an unknown aetiology that has a profound, but short-lasting effect upon the vision, and electrophysiological function of the eye.

Its anatomical presentation may only be mild to moderate, while visual changes may be quite severe. Symptoms usually consist of a blurring of vision, flashing lights, or black spots, which are described as fixed in position in contrast to the floating or movable spots ascribed to vitreous floaters. The visual acuity is often in the 20/50–20/70 range. Rarely it falls to a poor level such as 20/200–20/400. A mild afferent pupillary defect may be present and the vision usually recovers to normal within 2–12 weeks.

Observable yellow-white lesions are seen deep to the retina at the level of the retinal pigment epithelium. Ranging from 100–200 μ in diameter, these spots can rarely become as large as 1 disc diameter. They may be confused with AMPPE, but are usually discrete lesions and do not become confluent as in AMPPE. They usually appear as clusters of small discrete dots at the level of the retinal pigment epithelium. The macula is usually spared, with the largest focus of these small spots being in the peripapillary area and the mid-periphery. Vasculitis is not a prominent finding.

There is also a curious absence of anterior chamber inflammation. At most, a 1+ cell and flare is described, as well as a 1–2+ vitreous cellular reaction. Keratic precipitates are not described.

A fine granularity is noticed in the foveal area, which is described as a reddish excavation somewhat similar to that seen in solar retinopathy measuring

Acute multifocal placoid pigment epitheliopathy (AMPPE)	**Multiple evanescent white dot syndrome (MEWDS)**
Definition • Retinal pigment epithelial inflammation with secondary iridocyclitis	**Definition** • Discrete, small, focal, multiple exudates of the retinal pigment epithelium (RPE) combined with choriocapillaris, Bruch's membrane, and overlapping into neurosensory retina
Presentation • Acute • Nongranulomatous	**Presentation** • Yellow–white lesions deep to the retina at the level of the RPE • Occasional minimal iritis • Occasional minimal vitritis
Investigation • Fluorescein angiogram • Rule out systemic viral infection	**Investigation** • Electroretinography (ERG) • Electro-oculography (EOG)
Therapy • None	**Therapy** • Unknown aetiology • Nonspecific symptomatic treatment
Complications • Macular pigment alteration • Macular scarring	**Complications** • RPE pigment changes may persist • Usually vision returns to normal • Usually ERG and EOG return to normal
Prognosis • Good	**Prognosis** • Excellent

Table 7.6 Acute multifocal placoid pigment epitheliopathy (AMPPE).

Table 7.7 Multiple evanescent white dot syndrome (MEWDS).

50–75 μ. This granularity may be a disturbance of the retinal pigment epithelium, and in the early fluorescein angiographic stages, these lesions show focal hyperfluorescence in the RPE and may again be composed of smaller clusters of tiny dots or specks. They later may show as window defects in the RPE due to alteration or death of the cells in that layer. In late-phase angiograms, diffuse staining of the RPE and staining of the optic disc may be noted. Mild leakage of dye from the retinal and disc capillaries is observed. Interestingly, fluorescein angiographic changes may persist long after the white dots are no longer clinically apparent either by ophthalmoscopy or slit-lamp examination with a 60 or 90 dioptre lens. In the late resolution stages, a fluorescein angiogram usually reverts to normal, although a few focal punctate defects may be seen in the RPE as transmission lesions.

Electroretinographic (ERG) studies performed in several of the patients have shown that MEWDS has a profound effect on the retinal physiology. The photopic a-wave and b-wave amplitudes are decreased as well as the scotopic a-waves and b-waves. These ERG findings indicate a widespread retinal physiological involvement out of proportion to the seemingly small anatomical involvement of the retina and RPE with the clusters of tiny white dots. As the disease resolves, the ERG responses are noted to return to normal.

In the acute phase of the disease the electrooculogram (EOG) also shows moderate light to dark ratios that appear to correspond with the severity of the disease, reflecting a more severe RPE and photoreceptor abnormality than is often observed clinically. Once again, as with the electroretinograph, as the disease resolves the EOG also returns to normal. The aetiology of MEWDS is obscure. Since its clinical course appears to resolve as well as the seemingly profound ERG and EOG findings out of proportion to the clinical signs, it is presumed that it may be a consequence of a viral infection, similar to AMPPE. Several patients have been described as having a preceding flu-like illness. Chorioretinitis is observed in this disorder, but appears to be self-limited, which would reflect the development of antibodies to a virus or some other inflammatory agent. While the function of the RPE appears to be profoundly disturbed during the course of the disease, the cells apparently do survive intact and resume normal function, as reflected by the ERG and EOG. Residual scars and defects of the RPE are rare.

The differential diagnosis for MEWDS would include AMPPE, serpiginous choroidopathy, multifocal choroiditis, bird-shot retinopathy, and a nonspecific retinal pigment epitheliitis. All of these entities have an unknown aetiology in common and all have a profound and more severe effect on the electrophysiological function of the eye than indicated by the clinical signs. It has been suggested that most or all of these have a viral aetiology.

BACTERIAL INFECTIONS

A host of bacteria may cause severe extraocular and intraocular infections(**7.18–7.22**). Certain esoteric bacterial infections can also cause eye disease, both by infection and by allergy to exotoxin.

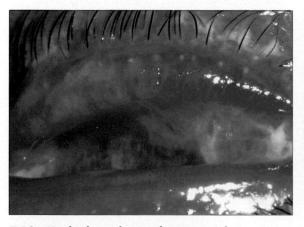

7.18 Marked purulence of gonococcal conjunctivitis in a 27-year-old white male.

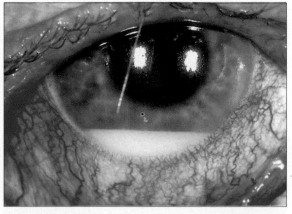

7.19 *Staphylococcus epidermidis* endophthalmitis following a cataract extraction.

BOTULISM

Botulism is a form of descending paralysis introduced by the exotoxin of the gram-positive anaerobic *Clostridium botulinum*. Usually ingested with contaminated food, the intestinal tract becomes overgrown by the organism. The toxin may also proliferate in a contaminated wound. Blurred vision and double vision usually accompany the acute gastrointestinal distress. Other ocular motility defects are less prominent, and ptosis, dilatation of the pupils, and reduced tear secretion may be present.

BRUCELLOSIS

Brucellosis, like tuberculosis and syphilis, may mimic any type of uveitis in the eye. It usually presents with optic nerve involvement, which is usually bilateral, papillary congestion, retrobulbar neuritis, frank papilloedema, and even atrophy. Many patients have a concomitant meningitis or arachnoiditis of the chiasm.

Uveitis has been reported, usually as a choroiditis with multiple nodular exudative areas with adjacent retinal oedema and haemorrhage.

Brucella has never been reported to be cultured from the eye. Presumed ophthalmitis from this organism may present with hypopyon progressing on to retinal detachment and ptosis.

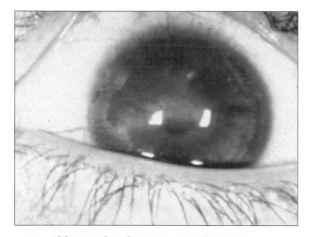

7.20 Phlyctenular disease secondary to blepharitis (Courtesy of Proctor Foundation Fellows Teaching Collection).

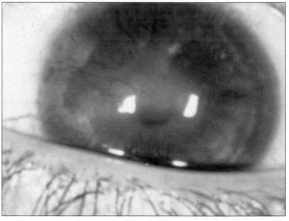

7.21 Enlargement showing the stromal changes following an initial epithelial disturbance in phlyctenular disease.

7.22 Episcleritis secondary to *Campylobacter*.

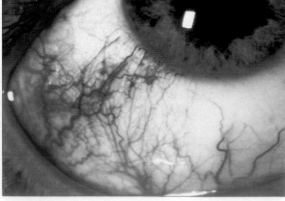

DIPHTHERIA

Diphtheria caused by *Corynebacterium diphtheriae* usually presents as an acute pharyngeal or skin infection followed weeks later by myocarditis with neuropathy. Neurological signs occur, and usually a light–near dissociation is described in which pupillary constriction to a nearby target is lost while constriction to light is maintained. While the aetiological basis for this neurological consequence is not known, it is probably a result of a peripheral neuropathy caused by the organism.

METASTATIC BACTERIAL ENDOPHTHALMITIS

Metastatic bacterial endophthalmitis is still a rare disease, but usually occurs with septicaemia, due today to immunosuppression and/or intravenous drug abuse. The patients in the former category usually include those with diabetes mellitus and those taking exogenous corticosteroids or immunosuppressives due to cancer treatment or organ transplant surgery. The latter category will be discussed in more detail in the chapter dealing with intravenous drug abuse.

CHLAMYDIAL INFECTIONS

Chlamydia is a gram-negative intracellular organism that shares characteristics of both bacteria and virions, but is different from both. The unique and biphasic life cycle differentiates this organism from all other microorganisms, and places it in an order of its own.

Chlamydia trachomatis, one of the two species in the one genus, is responsible for the eye disease of both trachoma and infectious venereal disease. While chlamydial infections are associated with increased antibody titres, reinfection is possible in both the ocular and genitourinary disease.

The most common manifestation of chlamydial infection is adult inclusion conjunctivitis with follicular hypertrophy, most pronounced in the inferior tarsal conjunctiva. Since this may be the presenting sign in Reiter's syndrome, it was thought for some time that Reiter's disease may be mediated by the autoimmune mechanism of postinfectious Chlamydia acquisition. While trachoma is currently more associated with disease in the Middle East, it is still seen in the United States, especially among Navajo Indians in the Southwest. It usually manifests as a superior tarsal follicular and papillary hypertrophy with end-stage scarring and secondary corneal opacification, entropion and trichiasis. Herbert's pits are small prominent excavated sites of inactive follicle formation in the superior limbus and may be diagnostic of previous trachoma infection.

HELMINTHIC DISEASES

CYSTICERCOSIS

The helminthic diseases include cysticercosis (*Taenia solium*), which manifests as either a free-floating cyst in the anterior chamber or posterior chamber or is subretinal in location. It may show a dense white dot in the centre, representing the invaginated scolex or head of the helminth, and can be treated by diathermy, cryotherapy or photocoagulation.

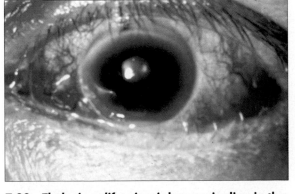

7.23 *Thelazia californiensis* **larva wiggling in the anterior chamber of eye** in a patient who acquired this infestation from a horse.

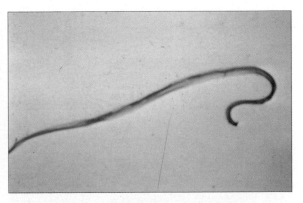

7.24 *Thelazia californiensis* extracted from the anterior chamber of the patient in **7.23**.

HYDATID DISEASE

Echinococcus or hydatid disease usually manifests with exophthalmos caused by the cestodes of the *Echinococcus*. While many human infections of this helminth remain silent and asymptomatic, the clinical manifestations are determined solely by the location of the cysts and their size. While they may occur in any of the systemic organs, the orbit represents only 1% of all systemic locations. Orbital cysts account for a high percentage of eye disease in the Middle East and in the United States. Subretinal, vitreous, and anterior chamber cysts have all been reported occasionally.

Treatment is usually excision of the cuticular membrane and contents from an orbital approach.

LOA LOA

Loa loa (**7.25**) is a helminth that is uncommon outside Africa. The systemic manifestations occur as a 'calabar' swelling, a hot pruritic swelling under the skin from 2–3 cm in size to many times this size. It may also occur as an arthritic change, an endomyocardial fibrosis, or meningoencephalitis. While the ocular manifestations are variable, most typically the worm is noted under the surface conjunctiva of the eye and causes itching, pain and irritation. Many local remedies are recommended, but surgical removal of the parasite is the definitive treatment.

ONCHOCERCIASIS

Onchocerciasis or river blindness occurs in both equatorial Africa and Central America, and is one of the leading causes of blindness in the world. The systemic manifestation is usually an infection under the skin from microfilaria, and pruritus is the earliest and most common sign.

Perivasculitis from the skin infection is one of the earliest skin changes and the ocular manifestations are secondary to the presence of both living and dead microfilaria in all coats of the eye manifesting as an inflammatory response. In the posterior segment, active motile microfilaria may be seen in the vitreous and retina without visible scarring, but these changes may also lead to large geographical areas of choroidal and retinal atrophy with severe vision loss. Vasculitis usually accompanies these changes in the posterior pole.

A newly developed drug, ivermectin, has revolutionized the treatment of onchocerciasis, and has been donated on a philanthropic basis to the countries in Africa that are affected. While ivermectin kills the microfilaria, it has no effect on the adult worms, so treatment must continue for up to 10 years until the adult helminths die.

SCHISTOSOMIASIS

Schistosomiasis is caused by the trematodes of the genus *Schistosoma*. Skin invasion by these helminths with a primary exposure causes mild transitory inflammatory itching at the site of penetration. Usually the bladder and ureters are principally involved, with cystitis being an early manifestation of systemic inflammation.

The ocular manifestations are usually a consequence of the urinary form of the disease and include urticaria, swelling and oedema of the eyelids. Systemic fever may also occur, and anterior nongranulomatous iridocyclitis has been reported.

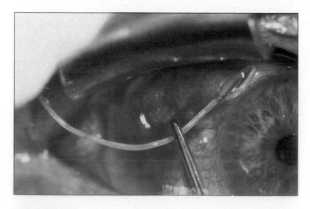

7.25 Loa loa being extracted from under the conjunctiva in a patient who had visited Africa and acquired this infestation. (Courtesy of Jonathan Belmont, MD.)

MYCOBACTERIAL INFECTIONS

TUBERCULOSIS

Mycobacterium tuberculosis can manifest itself in many types of ocular inflammations (**7.26–7.31, Table 7.8**).
- Tuberculous conjunctival granulomas are a cause of Parinaud's oculoglandular syndrome, and may cause systemic disease as well

- Phlyctenular keratitis and conjunctivitis are supposed hypersensitivity reactions to tubercular proteins.
- Tuberculous iridocyclitis occurs with and without associated corneal lesions.
- Panuveitis may be the most profound manifestation of the ocular-acquired form of the disease.
- Vasculitis may occur in the retina along with choroiditis either as focal choroidal tubercles or more diffuse inflammatory material under the retina.

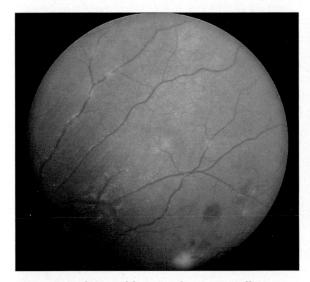

7.26 Vasculitis and haemorrhage as well as cotton wool exudation in a 14-year-old male from Tijuana, Mexico, with tuberculous choroiditis and retinitis.

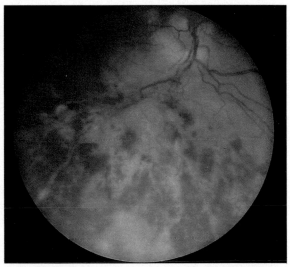

7.27 Marked retinal haemorrhage, vasculitis, and exudation in the same patient as in **7.26**.

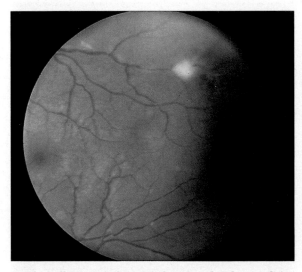

7.28 Fellow eye showing less involved vasculitis and retinal cotton wool exudation.

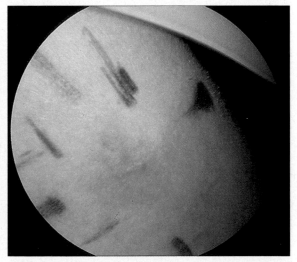

7.29 Marked swelling and over 10 mm of induration in the skin with intermediate purified protein derivative of tuberculin (PPD) in the patient in **7.26**.

Mycobacteria 1: tuberculosis

Definition
- Iridocyclitis, choroiditis, retinitis with vitritis

Presentation
- Usually choroiditis first
- Granulomatous

Investigation
- Sputum/bronchial lavage culture
- Tuberculin skin test
- Chest radiograph
- Erythrocyte sedimentation rate
- Medical consultation
- Serum lysozyme
- Human immunodeficiency virus test

Therapy
- Treat acute recurrent iridocyclitis with steroids
- Treat chronic iridocyclitis and choroiditis lesions with systemic steroids covered by antituberculous therapy (INH and rifampin)

Complications
- Variable

Prognosis
- Variable

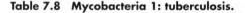

Table 7.8   Mycobacteria 1: tuberculosis.

- Tuberculous nodules may range in size from 0.25–0.5 inch disc diameter, may have either distinct or indistinct borders, and in Caucasian patients may simulate a malignant melanoma of the choroid. Nodules, whether located in the conjunctiva, iris, choroid, retina or optic nerve head, consist of the characteristic caseating necrosis: tubercles surrounded by a mononuclear infiltrate of cells.
- Inflammation may be diffuse and may affect all coats of the eye.

In contradistinction to sarcoidosis, which is a noncaseating granuloma, tuberculosis usually occurs as the necrotizing variety. Historically, it may be identified with acid-fast stains such as Ziehl–Neelsen or Fite stain and found in lesions of the retina, choroid, ciliary body, iris, cornea, conjunctiva, and orbit.

LEPROSY

Mycobacterium leprae (**7.32–7.43, Table 7.9**) is an unusual and exotic infection in the USA, but should nevertheless be considered a cause of uveitis for patients in the USA and UK. Native populations from China, Samoa, Hawaii, the Philippines, and the Sonoran province of Mexico may bring endemic leprosy with them. A prolonged period of contact is necessary to acquire the infection.

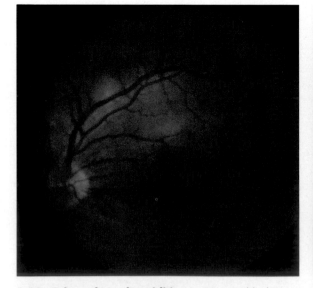

7.30 Tuberculous choroiditis in a 23-year-old white female airline hostess from the Philippines.

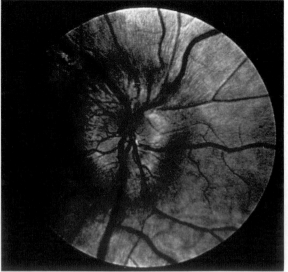

7.31 Papilloedematous changes in tuberculous meningitis in a 25-year-old white female.

The clinical manifestations of lepromatous uveitis differ considerably from the other mycobacteria (i.e. tuberculosis) in that *M. leprae* exclusively affects the anterior segment of the eye, preferring the cooler temperatures for its survival and multiplication.

Leprosy occurs in two distinct forms—lepromatous and tuberculoid—with an intermediate spectrum between them. The basic difference between these two forms depends upon the patient's intact or absent cell-mediated immunity.

- In the lepromatous form of the disease, which is diffuse and can involve many organs, profuse numbers of organisms are seen due to the lack of the patient's cell-mediated immunity.
- In the tuberculoid form cell-mediated immunity is intact and there is a localized form of the disease affecting one organ or one organ system only. Its predilection is for neural tissue, and only isolated organisms can be identified in histological specimens.

Patients who have leprosy may no longer feel the need to confine themselves to leprasaria and may be found in the general population as the Biblical view and old fashioned prejudices have disappeared or diminished in the Western world. A high index of suspicion for this type of infection must now be engendered in physicians in the USA because of the recent influx of Indochinese who come from areas where leprosy and tuberculosis are endemic.

Mycobacteria 2: leprosy

(Hansen's disease)

Definition
- Anatomical iridocyclitis only (predilection of organisms for cooler parts of the body)

Presentation
- Acute or chronic iridocyclitis
- Granulomatous or nongranulomatous

Investigation
- Anterior chamber tap (Fite stain or Ziehl–Neelsen stain)

Therapy
- Dapsone
- Rifampin
- Treat iridocyclitis with steroids after covering with antimicrobial

Complications
- Secluded pupil
- Corneal decompensation
- Cataract

Table 7.9   Mycobacteria 2: leprosy.

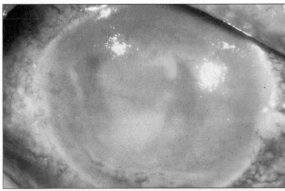

7.32   Profound lepromatous iridocyclitis obscuring all details of the anterior segment.

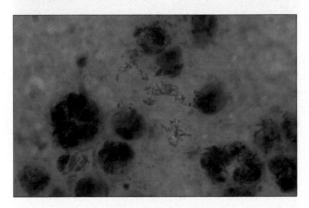

7.33   Aqueous aspirate of the patient in 7.32 demonstrating acid-fast bacilli with Fite stain.

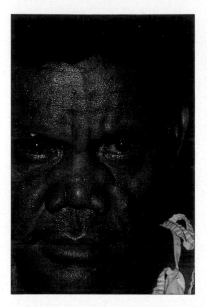

7.34 A patient with acute lepromatous 'leonine facies' due to resorbed nasal cartilage. Note the absence of distal pinky digit due to loss from lepromatous leprosy.

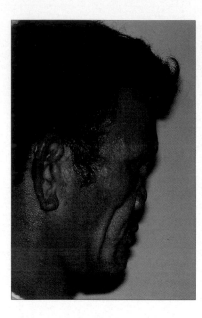

7.35 Profile of the patient in 7.34 showing marked resorption of nasal cartilage due to his lepromatous infection.

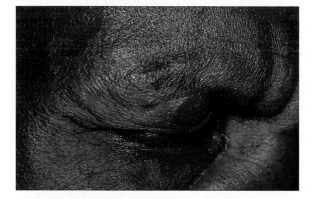

7.36 Subepidermal nodule in lepromatous leprosy.

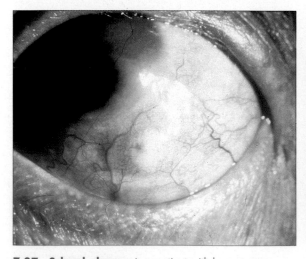

7.37 Scleral abscess in a patient with lepromatous leprosy and iridocyclitis.

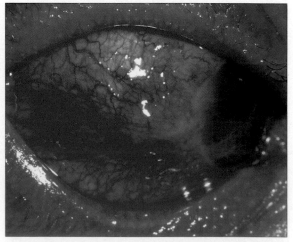

7.38 Marked conjunctival and episcleral erythema surrounding lepromatous nodule on the sclera.

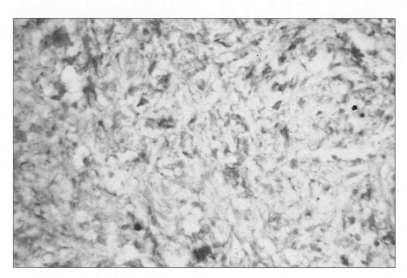

7.39 Ziehl–Neelsen stain of sclera demonstrating a multitude of acid-fast bacilli indicative of lepromatous-type leprosy infection.

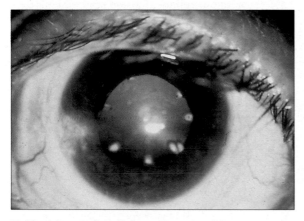

7.40 Iris pearls, which are Koeppe nodules composed of active leprosy organisms surrounded by fibrous tissue.

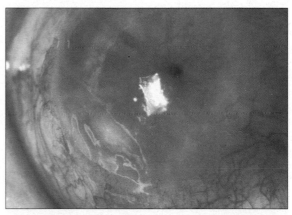

7.41 Corneal erosion, drying, iridocyclitis and seclusion of pupil in a patient with an active leprosy kerato-uveitis.

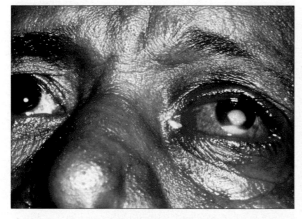

7.42 A 32-year-old patient with lepromatous leprosy with corneal ulcer, hypopyon, madarosis, and dacryocystitis.

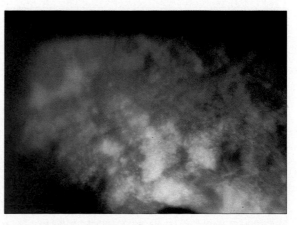

7.43 Yellow cheesy nodular lepromata of leprosy infection, superior iris.

FUNGAL INFECTIONS

PRESUMED OCULAR HISTOPLASMOSIS

Presumed ocular histoplasmosis (POHS, **7.44–7.51, Table 7.10**) is a disease of young adults that was originally described in the 1960s and now is very commonly diagnosed in areas where *Histoplasma capsulatum* is endemic. It is also seen in countries where histoplasmosis is not known to occur. Currently about 3 million patients have positive *Histoplasma* skin tests in the USA. Of these, an estimated 4% have peripheral or peripapillary scarring

in the retina. Subretinal neovascular membranes that haemorrhage cause blindness in this disorder and account for a considerable proportion of young people who have a central loss of vision.

The clinical features of POHS are serous and haemorrhagic detachment of the macula, peripheral and peripapillary 'punched-out' scars, and a peripapillary depigmentation or scarring. These signs constitute the classical triad of POHS. It is important to observe that the anterior chamber and vitreous are clear of cells in this disease.

Active disease may occur around peripapillary scarring with subretinal fluid extending underneath the macular zone. This may cause metamorphopsia

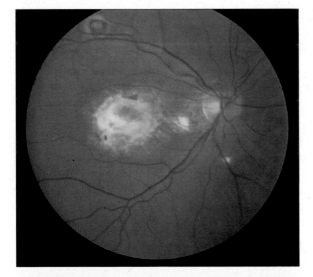

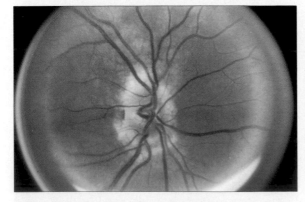

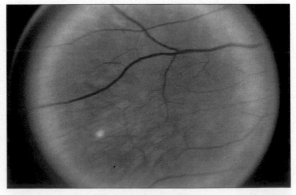

7.44 Scarring of retinal pigment epithelium in a 24-year-old white female with histoplasmic choroiditis.

7.45 Typical peripapillary depigmentation, which forms part of presumed ocular histoplasmosis in the eye.

7.46 'Peripheral punched-out lesion' as part of the triad of presumed ocular histoplasmosis.

and reduced central vision, but the true loss of central vision occurs from subretinal neovascular membrane. Subretinal neovascular membrane may occur in the absence of the full triad of this disease, and some clinicians consider that these patients have histoplasmosis until proven otherwise. However, other diseases in young people can cause subretinal neovascular membrane and these include angioid streaks, choroidal rupture, Fuch's spot, other 'thinnings' of Bruch's membrane, Ehlers–Danlos syndrome, sickle cell anaemia, and Paget's disease.

The aetiology of most cases of POHS remains unproven since many of these patients will not have documented pulmonary histoplasmosis. However, in the USA, the organism is endemic in the Mississippi, Ohio, and Missouri River valleys. It is assumed that a systemic fungaemia developing early may cause a mild upper respiratory infection, and this may seed to the eyes and/or central nervous system.

Therapy is indicated in POHS for a suspected systemic fungaemia, especially in the absence of pulmonary *Histoplasma* infection. Photocoagulation appears to offer benefit in eliminating subretinal neovascular membrane, especially with krypton laser in and about the fovea. Other clinicians favour corticosteroids in addition to argon photocoagulation when subretinal neovascular membrane can be established beyond question by fluorescein angiography and if the lesion is in a treatable area outside the capillary-free zone of the fovea. When a patient has a subretinal neovascular membrane in one eye and small atrophic areas are found either by clinical examination or fluorescein angiography in the macula of the second eye, the patient has a 20–25% chance

Presumed ocular histoplasmosis (POHS)

Definition
- Triad: Peripapillary pigment change
  Peripheral 'punched out' lesions
  Subretinal neovascular membrane under macula

Presentation
- Subretinal neovascular membrane in the macular region
- Peripheral 'punched-out' lesions
- Nongranulomatous choroiditis

Investigation
- *Histoplasma* skin test
- Chest radiograph
- HLA B7 (if macula is involved)

Therapy
- Vigorous treatment of symptoms of metamorphopsia with high-dose, short-course, systemic steroids may be helpful
- Photocoagulation of macula-threatening lesions may be of benefit

Complications
- Macular scarring
- Loss of sensorineural vision

Prognosis
- Good if no lesion in or near the macula
- Ominous to poor if a lesion is present in the macula due to recurrent activity

Table 7.10   Presumed ocular histoplasmosis (POHS).

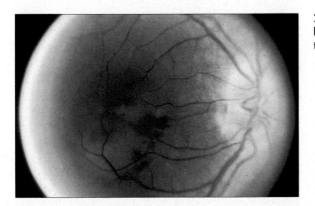

7.47   Acute subretinal neovascular membrane haemorrhage in a patient with the third component of the triad of presumed ocular histoplasmosis syndrome.

of developing macular disease from subretinal neo-vascular membrane in the fellow eye. Attention should be paid to early recognition of metamor-phopsia and other visual complaints in the fellow eye for possible intervention with krypton, or yellow dye laser photocoagulation. Some of these eyes with "pora foveal" subretinal membranes may be so suc-cessfully treated with lasers that their vision may improve from legal blindness to useful or even good vision.

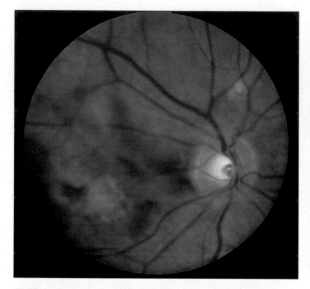

7.48 Extensive subretinal haemorrhage from subretinal neovascular membrane in a patient with presumed ocular histoplasmosis. Note the peripheral punched-out lesions superior to the optic papilla.

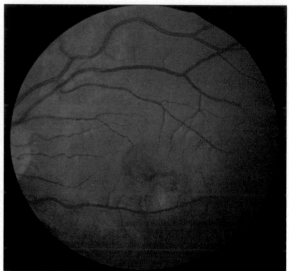

7.49 Small but devastating leakage and haemorrhage from subretinal neovascular membrane in a 20-year-old white female with presumed ocular histoplasmosis. The location of this subretinal neovascular membrane may make this patient an appropriate candidate for laser treatment.

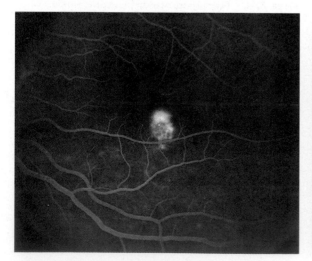

7.50 Fluorescein angiogram of the patient in 7.49 demonstrating the slightly eccentric location of this subretinal neovascular membrane from the fovea itself, making this patient a candidate for laser treatment.

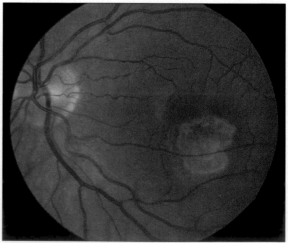

7.51 Fundus of the patient in 7.49 showing laser treatment and obliteration of neovascular membrane in this 20-year-old white female who had a return of 20/30 vision in this eye with an only slightly disabling macular scotoma.

COCCIDIOIDOMYCOSIS

San Joachim Valley Fever (**7.52, Table 7.11**) or 'Valley fever,' is caused by *Coccidioides immitis*. It is endemic to the southwestern region of the USA, the northwestern region of Mexico, Central America, and Venezuela. Ocular involvement was first described at the turn of the century in a patient with disseminated disease with both corneal and conjunctival involvement.

The infection usually begins as a pulmonary infestation and may be present without symptoms in up to 75% of cases. When manifest, a bronchial pneumonia is most common and the prognosis is good. Up to 5% of all patients with manifest pulmonary infection develop disseminated disease elsewhere.

The intraocular findings include iridocyclitis, often of a granulomatous nature, and multiple yellow-white chorioretinal lesions 0.1–0.5 disc diameter in size, often having a pigmented border and only occasionally showing creamy/runny retinal exudates. Most of the retinal lesions look like 'acute' histo lesions.

The usual treatment is intravenous amphotericin B. Extraocular lesions may also occur in the lid, orbit and conjunctiva, and may be associated with a phlyctenular conjunctivitis and/or episcleritis.

Coccidioidomycosis

Definition
- San Joachim Valley Fever
- Southwestern USA

Presentation
- Primary bronchopneumonia
- Phlyctenular conjunctivitis
- Episcleral, conjunctival, lid lesions
- Multiple yellow-white chorioretinal lesions with pigmented border
- 'Punched-out' peripheral lesions

Investigation
- Chest radiograph
- Biopsy of skin, lid, conjunctival lesion
- Complement-fixing antibodies
- Immunodiffusion for IgM, IgG

Therapy
- Amphotericin B (intravenous, intrathecal)
- Steroids

Prognosis
- Disease can be fatal

Table 7.11 Coccidioidomycosis.

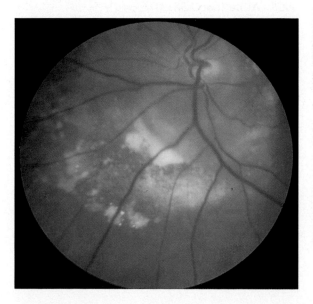

7.52 Coccidiomycosis infection of the optic nerve and choroid in a patient with San Joachim Valley Fever and meningitis.

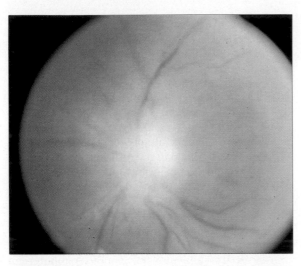

7.53 Vitreous fluff ball surrounded by less intense vitritis in a patient with a *Candida* endophthalmitis secondary to intravenous drug abuse.

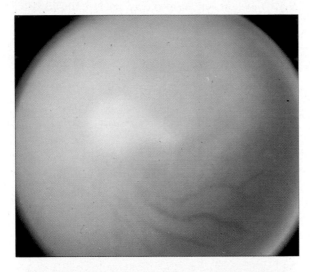

7.54 Another patient with a vitreous fluff ball adjacent to the optic nerve head with a more intense vitreous involvement secondary to *Candida* endophthalmitis due to intravenous drug abuse.

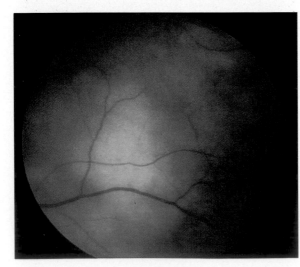

7.55 Acute choroiditis in a young male with blastomycosis and encephalitis.

SPIROCHAETAL INFECTIONS

SYPHILIS

Syphilis (**7.56–7.63, Table 7.12**), at one time over-diagnosed if not misdiagnosed as a common cause of uveitis, became rare when brought under antimicrobial control. Recently, due to the worldwide resurgence of veneral disease in general and AIDS in particular, there is a fully documented increase in syphilitic ocular disease. Syphilis must therefore still be considered in the differential diagnosis of uveitis.

The fluorescent treponemal antibody absorption test (FTA–ABS) is the most sensitive indicator for syphilis infection. Occasionally, when syphilis has been only partially treated or in cases of central nervous system syphilis, the FTA–ABS is positive and the Venereal Disease Research Laboratory test (VDRL) is negative.

Congenital syphilis is usually manifested by the 'salt-and-pepper fundus' inflammation of the retinal pigment epithelium, with its concomitant typical corneal lesions and pale optic nerve.

Acquired syphilis causes various types of ocular inflammation including iris nodules, iridocyclitis, which may be severe and unresponsive to corticosteroid

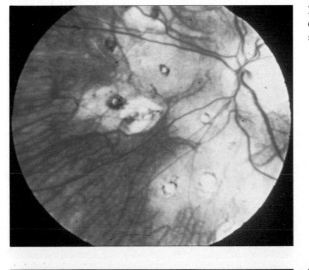

7.56 Marked retinal pigment epithelial disturbance in an 8-year-old patient with congenital syphilis.

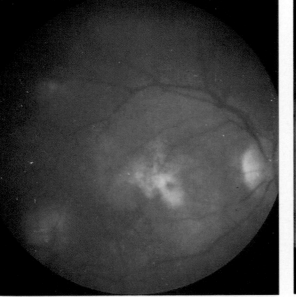

7.57 Choroiditis secondary to late tertiary syphilis with reactivation as uveitis in a 68-year-old Algerian female.

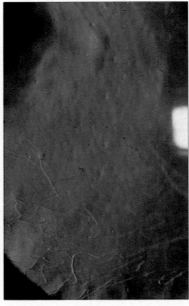

7.58 Ghost vessels indicative of inactive interstitial keratitis in a 24-year-old white male who had previously had active primary and secondary syphilis.

therapy, and in some cases, large keratic precipitates. An indolent progressive type of iridocyclitis should alert the clinician to the possibility of this newly resurgent disease. Papillitis may be the manifestation of systemic syphilis infection. Diffuse chorioretinitis, choroiditis, and particularly vasculitis, are additional complications that may occur later in the disease or may be clinical signs indicating steroid-unresponsive uveitis.

Any or all of these ocular inflammatory signs may be associated with the skin lesions of secondary syphilis, including a maculopapular rash, which is usually found on the palms and the soles.

These ocular forms of syphilis gradually worsen and progress from initial iridocyclitis to the whole spectrum of syphilitic eye disease, and are often accompanied by vasculitis of the posterior pole.

Current treatment suggests systemic therapy of 24 million units of intravenous penicillin; the ocular inflammation is treated with steroids. Penicillamine is advocated by some authorities to enhance penicillin absorption. A worldwide increase in syphilis accompanied the emergence of HIV. The acquisition of syphilis increases the risk of developing HIV infection and AIDS and there are many reported instances of their concurrence.

Syphilis

Definition
- Acute or chronic infection

Presentation
- Presents as anything (mimicker as with sarcoidosis)
- Granulomatous
- Chronic, even in conjunctivitis
- Mucous membrane secondary rash
- Iritis and nodules (roseata and papulata)
- Retinal vasculitis
- Choroiditis

Investigation
- Venereal Disease Reference Laboratory test (VDRL); rapid plasma reagin test (RPR); response to treatment (RST)
- Fluorescent treponemal antibody absorption test (FTA–ABS (specific tests)
- MHA–TP (specific tests)
- Lumbar puncture
- Human immunodeficiency virus (HIV) test also necessary
- Medical consultation

Therapy
- Systemic penicillin; current regimen 24 million units intravenously
- Treat ocular inflammation with steroids

Complications
- Cataracts
- Glaucoma
- Macular scarring
- Optic nerve dysfunction and scarring
- Phthisis

Prognosis
- Variable
- Sometimes refractory to full treatment

Table 7.12 Syphilis.

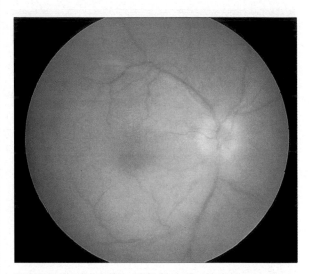

7.59 Acute retinitis with foci of exudative precipitates in a 27-year-old white male stockbroker with papillitis and retinal infection secondary to tertiary syphilis, who is also HIV-positive.

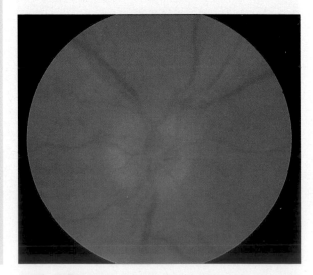

7.60 Fellow eye demonstrating papillitis changes.

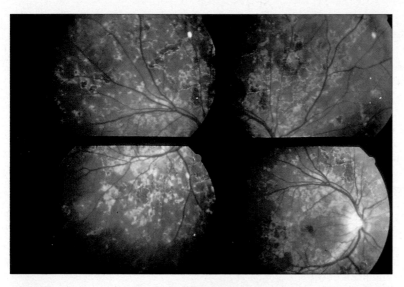

7.61   A 27-year-old white male with tertiary syphilis with profound retinal pigment epithelial disturbance. (Courtesy of Howard Schatz, MD)

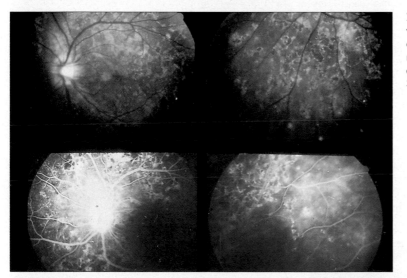

7.62   Same patient as in 7.61 with accompanying fluorescein angiographic changes highlighting the marked retinal pigment epithelial disturbance. (Courtesy of Howard Schatz, MD)

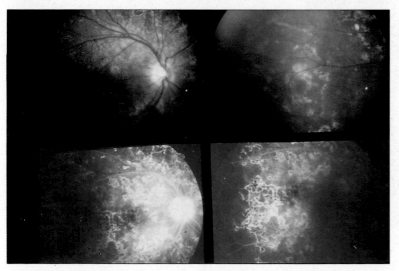

7.63   Fellow eye of the same 27-year-old white male shown in 7.61 with the fluorescein angiographic highlights of this very profound retinal pigment epithelial change. (Courtesy of Howard Schatz, MD)

PARASITIC INFECTIONS

TOXOPLASMOSIS

Toxoplasmosis (**7.64–7.73, Table 7.13**) is an infection of an obligate intracellular protozoan parasite and may represent the most common form of posterior uveitis in the developed world. *Toxoplasma gondii* is ubiquitous in the warm-blooded animal kingdom: the parasite undergoes the sexual stage reproduction in the intestinal mucosal epithelium in the cat, its primary host. Oocysts shed by the cat in faeces are then ingested by intermediate hosts such as rodents and birds, which are caught by cats again, therefore perpetuating the life cycle, and who then serve as vectors to carnivorous animals and to grazing herbivorous animals. Man then eats the flesh of the herbivores to liberate the *Toxoplasma* organisms. Infection may therefore be acquired by the consumption of raw or improperly cooked meat.

Of the systemic varieties of toxoplasmosis, approximately 1% demonstrate ocular lesions. The vast majority of patients seen by the ophthalmologist probably have congenitally acquired disease that reactivates later in life.

The organism resides in the long term in neural tissue, and may remain dormant for long periods of time, but may reactivate in later life giving the impression of a new infection. Fetal brain and ocular tissues are especially susceptible to long-term parasitization. Therefore affected neonates usually manifest healed scars, which are susceptible to recurrent inflamation at a later time.

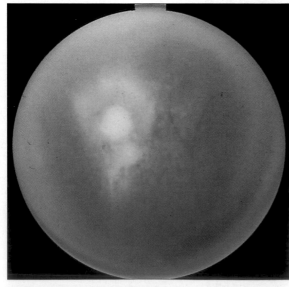

7.64 Acute toxoplasmic retinitis in focus contiguous to a previous scarred lesion.

Systemic toxoplasmosis may manifest itself in four forms:
- An exanthematous eruption due to a skin vasculitis, which resembles rickettsial disease in appearance: this rare entity is the most fatal form of the disease.

Toxoplasmosis
Definition
• Acute retinitis
Presentation
• Retinitis or retinochoroiditis
• Granulomatous
Investigation
• *Toxoplasma*
• Sabin–Feldman dye test
• Fluorescent antibody test for *Toxoplasma*
• Enzyme-linked immunosorbent assay (ELISA) test for *Toxoplasma*
• Aqueous antibodies (as a proportion of serum antibodies) in unusual presentation
Therapy
• Vigorous for the lesion:
–if threatening the macula, the maculopapillary bundle, the optic nerve
–if there is severe endophthalmitis
–if there is macular oedema secondary to lesions superior to the macula
• Pyrimethamine (Daraprim®) and sulfa in combination
• Can use sulfa alone
• Can use tetracycline (minocycline)
• Can use systemic or periocular clindamycin
• Concurrent systemic steroids
• Never start steroids before antimicrobials
• Avoid periocular steroids alone
• Avoid systemic steroids without antimicrobial coverage
Complications
• Secondary anterior uveitis with posterior synechiae
• Secondary cataract
• Secondary glaucoma
• Retinal scarring (macula)
• Traction retinal detachment
Prognosis
• Fair to poor if the lesion is near the macula
• Recurrent lesions may affect the foveal region
• Excellent if only a peripheral lesion (may require no treatment)

Table 7.13 Toxoplasmosis.

- A lymphadenopathic infection, which may resemble a heterophil-negative 'mononucleosis' syndrome, and includes fever, malaise, lymphadenopathy, myalgias, and perhaps a mild elevation of liver enzymes.
- A meningoencephalitic syndrome, which is associated with a higher frequency of eye involvement than the more common lymphadenopathic form and usually manifests itself as seizures, fever, and profound central nervous system signs.
- A congenital syndrome, which is the least common and most severe form and is signified by the

'Sabin' tetrad of seizures, hydrocephalus, retinochoroiditis, and cerebral calcifications.

Toxoplasmosis is initially a pure retinitis and forms a retinochoroiditis only secondarily. This aspect of *Toxoplasma* infection distinguishes it from the other 'chorioretinitides.'

The clinical signs of toxoplasmic retinochoroiditis include the stigmata of 'granulomatous' uveitis. Usually mutton-fat keratic precipitates are present, an intense anterior chamber reaction and an outpouring of cells into the vitreous, especially over the white inflammatory focus of the retina. Older lesions

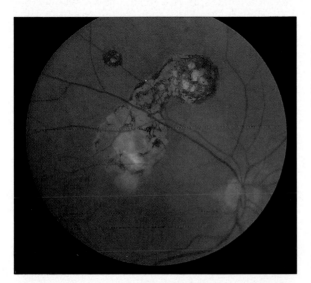

7.65 Interesting helicoid-shaped, progressive recurrent toxoplasmic retinitis, which began supratemporal to the optic nerve head and progressed in an intermittent fashion, reactivating in an inferiorly direction until its final focus of acute activation seen here is kissing into the fovea. The patient's resultant vision was 20/30, but ultimately it was lost to further reactivation in the fovea itself.

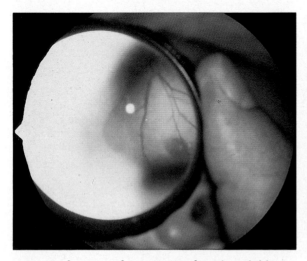

7.66 Roth's spot of acute toxoplasmic retinitis in a patient immunocompromised with Hodgkin's disease who also developed toxoplasmic meningitis and ultimately died.

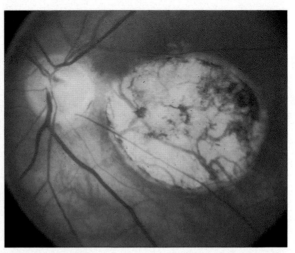

7.67 Classical congenital toxoplasmosis lesion, which is inactive but had obliterated the macula in this 12-year-old youngster.

are usually pigmented by retinal pigment epithelium hypertrophy and accompanied by local retinal vasculitis. Resolution of the lesion in the retina is marked by a pigmented scar.

Reactivation usually occurs in proximity to an older lesion in a so-called satellite focus. Vitreous membranes may occur when the gel is infiltrated by an intense outpouring of cells and may lead to traction retinal detachment. Retinal breaks are not uncommon in severe cases. Focal retinal necrosis may occur.

The diagnosis of *Toxoplasma* infection is still a clinical one, but it is corroborated by the presence of antibodies in the serum of the patient. These antibodies may be assayed by immunofluorescence, Sabin–Feldman dye test, haemagglutination or the new microtitre enzyme-linked immunosorbent assay (ELISA) test. A positive IgM level indicates previous exposure to the organism, but rising titres of IgG are indicative of current or recurrent infection. Patients with acquired systemic infection usually have titres over 1:256, while patients with the pure ocular form of the disease may have antibodies only to a 1:1 dilution. For this reason, it is often necessary to specify to the laboratory that the patient's serum should be run undiluted since many laboratories routinely dilute all specimens to a base level of 1:4 or 1:8.

The treatment of the infection includes antiprotozoals: pyrimethamine, sulfadiazine or triple sulfa and steroids. Pyrimethamine and the sulfas work synergistically, and it is appropriate to initiate these before the inclusion of steroid if either the macula or optic papilla are threatened since the local immunosuppression caused by the steroid may cause further damage to the sensitive neural tissues. Suppression of the bone marrow may occur with the use of pyrimethamine, and monitoring of the platelet and leukocyte count is essential. Folinic acid, a folic acid antagonist, can be given orally to prevent the marrow suppression.

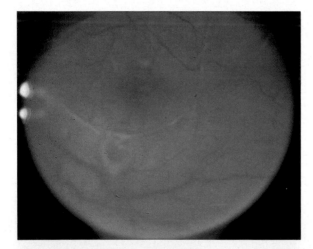

7.68 Tiny focus of active toxoplasmic retinitis in the macula that would mark vitreous inflammation with veils in the vitreous.

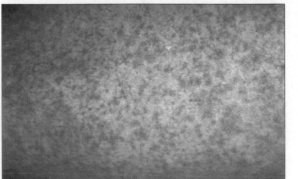

7.69 Extensive maculopapular eruption of the skin in toxoplasmic vasculitis. This cutaneous manifestation of toxoplasmosis resembles Rocky Mountain spotted fever.

Clindamycin has been shown to be an effective anti-protozoal, both orally and by sub-Tenon's injection. The former method has been shown to cause a pseudomembranous colitis, which can be therapeutically avoided (doxycycline), while the latter may be complicated by optic neuropathy. Minocycline is also advocated by some authorities as an alternative treatment. A very peripheral toxoplasmic 'hot spot' may not require treatment if the patient's immune system is intact and the essential visual structures (macula, disc) are not threatened. Toxoplasmosis is reported as an opportunistic infection in patients with AIDS.

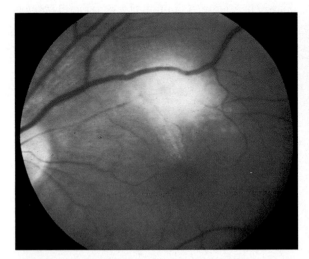

7.70 Acute focus of toxoplasmic retinitis in a patient who visited a mink farm and acquired the infection, presenting with a fever of unknown origin, lymphadenopathy, and sudden loss of vision.

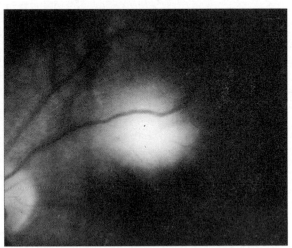

7.71 Fluorescein angiogram of the patient in 7.70 demonstrating that the toxoplasmic infection is localized exclusively to the retina and has not yet involved the retinal pigment epithelium.

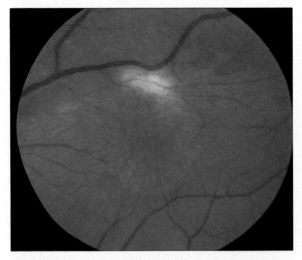

7.72 Fluorescein angiogram of the patient in 7.70 showing healing of the lesion without acute retinal or vitreous involvement, but demonstrating a marked fibrosis in the internal membrane of the retina and change in the retinal pigment epithelium.

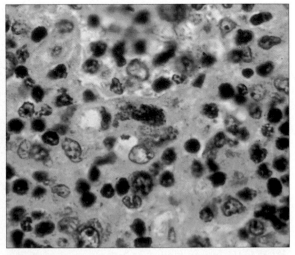

7.73 Axillary lymph node of the patient in 7.70 demonstrating toxoplasmosis cyst formation.

OCULAR TOXOCARIASIS

Toxocara canis infection (**7.75–7.77, Table 7.14**) occurs in children and its most frequent clinical sign is leukocoria. This clinical entity may often be confused with retinoblastoma and due to the potentially profound significance of misdiagnosis, very careful attention should be paid to the clinical signs and symptoms of children who present with this entity. Toxocariasis was first described in 1950 and is now recognized in three forms:

* A diffuse endophthalmitis.
* A macular retinal choroidal granuloma, often with a scar, which extends to the optic nerve head.
* A peripheral retinal choroidal granuloma.

The *Toxocara canis* is a common ascarid and is found in up to 50% of otherwise healthy dogs. The prevalence of human exposure as evidenced by a positive serology is less than 10% of the population.

Ocular toxocariasis is almost always unilateral, although very rarely bilateral cases are reported. It is unusual for it to occur after 12 years of age. Boys are affected more frequently than girls. Often there is a history of pica in children who become affected. It is of interest that visceral larval migrans, which is the systemic dermal variety of this disease, does not usually have the ocular manifestations associated with it, and vice versa. Approximately 2% of all patients diagnosed as having ocular toxocariasis have evidence of underlying visceral larval migrans, which is often characterized by fever, hepatosplenomegaly, and a high degree of eosinophilia, which seldom affects the eye. However, when an acute toxocariasis affects the eye, eosinophils may be isolated from the anterior chamber by paracentesis, while the peripheral blood profile is usually negative.

The ELISA for toxocariasis, is available through most state laboratories or the Center for Disease Control in Atlanta. A dilution of 1:8 for larval antigen

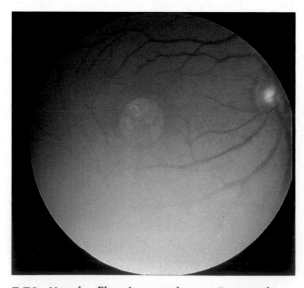

7.74 Macular fibrosis secondary to *Entamoeba histolytica* infection of the eye in a 42-year-old engineer from Mexico City.

Ocular toxocariasis
Definition
• Acute endophthalmitis
• Inactive, usually white, elevated scar on the retina with cicatrix leading to optic papilla
Presentation
• Endophthalmitis
• Inactive uveitis
• Scar from peripheral lesion to optic papilla
• Traction retinal detachment
• Granulomatous
Investigation
• Enzyme-linked immunosorbent assay (ELISA) for *Toxocara*
• Vitreous aspiration with ELISA
• Erythrocyte sedimentation rate
• Complete blood count
• AC tap for eosinophils (B scan for calcification)
Therapy
• Periocular steroids
• Systemic steroids during active period
• Antihelminths contraindicated
Complications
• Cataract
• Macular scarring
• Glaucoma
• Retinal detachment
Prognosis
• Poor if macula involved
• Poor if endophthalmitis is present
• If peripheral, prognosis is good with treatment of the severe phases of inflammation
• Once case is quiet, intraocular surgery is well tolerated for retinal attachment

Table 7.14 Ocular toxocariasis.

is considered positive and may help in diagnosing over 90% of cases. An ELISA performed on the aqueous humour is even more sensitive, especially when eosinophilia may be prominent. However, skin tests are considered unreliable because there is considerable cross-reaction with other types of ascarid and many healthy persons test positively even in the absence of any larval infection.

While medical treatment of ocular toxocariasis is generally unsatisfactory since antihelminth preparations release a burden of antigen which consume the eye in immunological reaction, suppression of the reaction with steroids is preferable. Recent reports demonstrate some structural improvement with vitrectomy surgery when the disease becomes chronic and inactive.

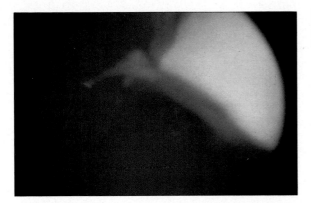

7.75 An 8-year-old white male with acute *Toxocara* infestation under the retina with abscess formation, exudation, and overlying vitreous cells.

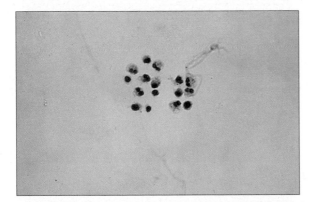

7.76 Eosinophils isolated from aqueous humour of the patient in **7.75**.

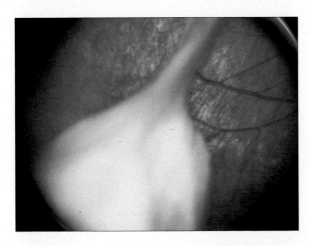

7.77 A 14-year-old patient with a peripheral organized *Toxocara canis*, but inactive abscess in the peripheral retina.

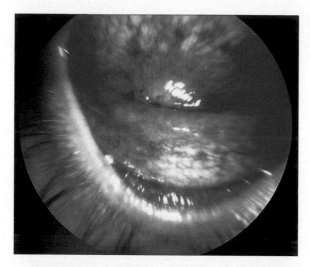

7.78 Marked epibulbar and conjunctival erythema in chemosis from Rocky Mountain spotted fever.

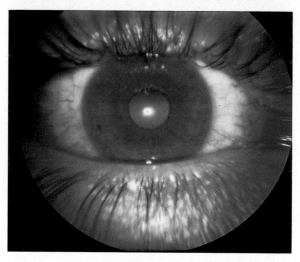

7.79 Synechiae and anterior chamber inflammation in a patient with iritis secondary to Rocky Mountain spotted fever.

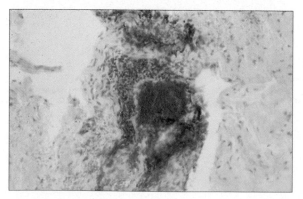

7.80 Conjunctival biopsy showing a necrotizing vasculitis secondary to Rocky Mountain spotted fever.

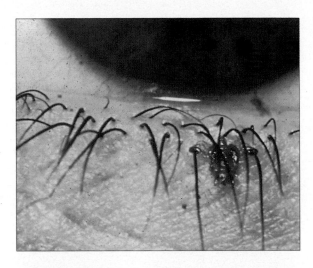

7.81 A *Phthirus pubis* extracted from eyelid of a patient in an emergency room.

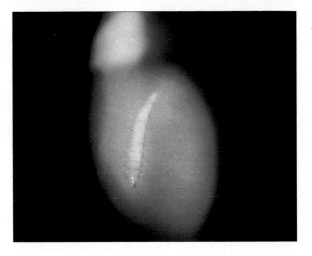

7.82 Botfly larva visualized in the vitreous of a patient who had been camping in Sierra Nevada and acquired this infestation. (Courtesy of Michael Goldbaum, MD.)

8.
Inflammatory and Autoimmune Diseases of Unknown Aetiology

BEHÇET'S DISEASE

Behçet's disease (**8.1–8.12, Table 8.1**) is characterized by three primary components:
- Iridocyclitis (historically with hypopyon).
- Aphthous lesions in the mouth.
- Ulceration of the genitalia.

Behçet's disease

Definition
- A systemic vasculitis with multi organ presentation

Presentation
- Iridocyclitis
- Retinitis
- Choroiditis
- Vasculitis
- Granulomatous

Investigation
- HLA B5, HLA Bw51
- Antibody test with guinea–pig lip
- Medical consultation
- Fluorescein angiogram
- Questionable skin puncture test (Behçetine test)

Therapy
- Intensive local systemic steroids
- Periocular steroids
- Low-dose chronic local or systemic steroids in chronic cases
- Consider immunosuppressive agents, especially chlorambucil, if retinal vasculitis present
- Cyclosporin

Complications
- Cataract
- Glaucoma
- Retinal necrosis
- Optic atrophy
- Phthisis bulbi

Prognosis
- Usually poor once eyes involved
- Blindness 3.3 years after initial eye manifestations

Table 8.1 Behçet's disease.

Erythema nodosum, arthropathy, and thrombophlebitis often accompany these manifestations, but the ocular symptoms may be the most important and serious manifestations of the disease. The frequency of ocular manifestations is 70–85%. Central nervous system involvement, most often due to necrotizing vasculitis, may be the most protean manifestation of the disease leading to death. The underlying disease mechanism in all organ systems is an occlusive vasculitis.

Although the most common ocular symptom is anterior uveitis, often with hypopyon, the presence of necrotizing peripheral occlusive vasculitis in the fundus is well known and often obscured by the severity of the anterior reaction. It is important to be familiar with the full spectrum of disease presentation because the ophthalmologist may be the first physician to encounter the patient with Behçet's disease.

Current treatment includes steroids and immunosuppressives, chlorambucil, azathioprine, cyclosporin, hydroxychloroquine and colchicine.

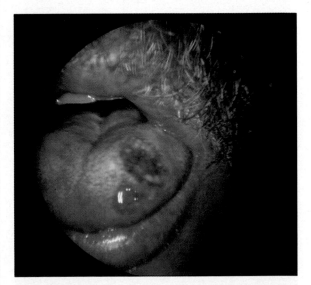

8.1 Aphthous ulceration on the tongue in a 24-year-old male with Behçet's disease. Note the active crater with haemorrhage in the adjacent healed aphthous ulcer next to it.

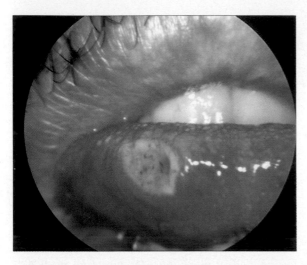

8.2 Deep crater aphthous ulcer on the tongue in a young male with Behçet's disease.

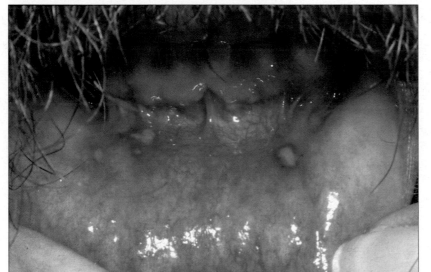

8.3 Two acute, tender and painful aphthous ulcers on the buccal mucosa.

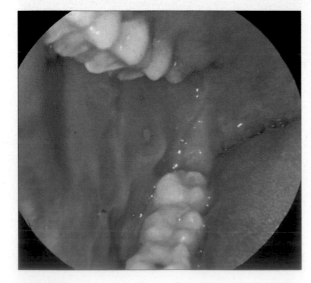

8.4 Buccal mucosa deep toward the pharynx demonstrating acute aphthous ulceration.

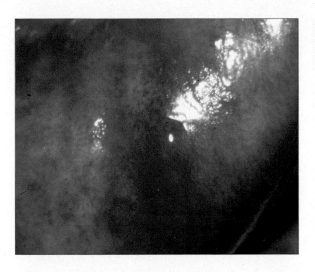

8.5 Healed aphthous ulcer on the buccal mucosa demonstrating scar tissue formation indicative of the underlying necrosing vasculitis, which is the hallmark of this disease histologically.

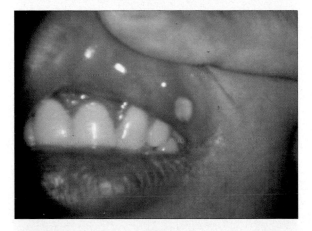

8.6 Healing aphthous lesion on the upper buccal mucosa.

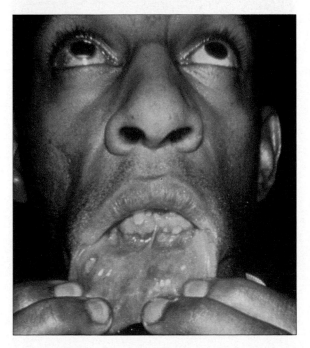

8.7 Classical presentation of a patient with multiple aphthous ulcerations of the buccal mucosa. Note the hypopyon and the inflamed right eye. (Courtesy of Wills Eye Hospital.)

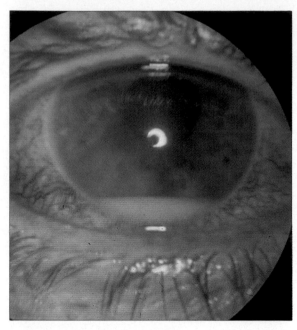

8.8 Hypopyon presentation in a 28-year-old white male with Behçet's iridocyclitis.

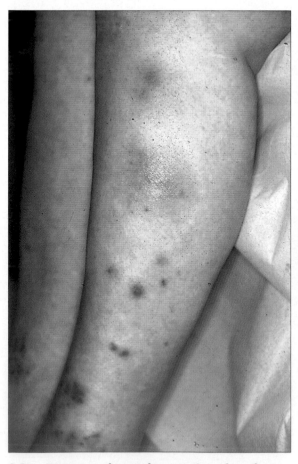

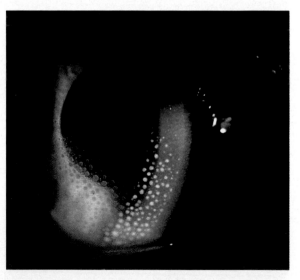

8.9b Acute iridocyclitis with large mutton-fat keratic precipitates in a patient with Behçet's iridocyclitis. Marked retinal vasculitis in retina, showing the typical presentation indicative of the underlying histological vasculitis present in all organ systems in Behçet's disease.

8.9a Acute maculopapular eruption of erythema nodosum typical of Behçet's disease presentation.

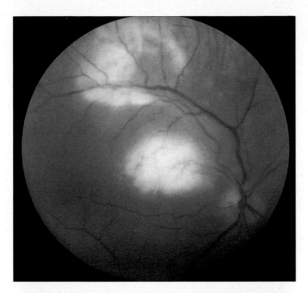

8.10 Acute retinal necrosis as a consequence of retinal vasculitis with Behçet's disease.

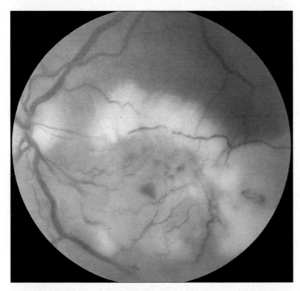

8.11 Profound macular surrounding retinal vasculitis leading to retinal necrosis in a patient with Behçet's disease who also had concurrent central nervous system vasculitis leading ultimately to a neurological death in this patient.

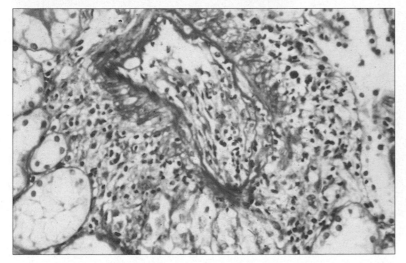

8.12 Histological picture of engorged and thrombosed vasculitic area of kidney in patient with Behçet's vasculitis.

VOGT–KOYANAGI–HARADA SYNDROME

Vogt–Koyanagi–Harada syndrome (**8.13–8.25, Table 8.2**) is the clinical brother of sympathetic ophthalmia. This panuveitis affects the iris, ciliary body, and choroid, and may manifest all of the same clinical signs as sympathetic ophthalmia.

Vogt–Koyanagi–Harada syndrome appears to be an autoimmune reaction to melanin or uveal pigment since the ocular and the central nervous system (uveoencephalitis) signs occur where melanosomes are present, as in the chorda tympani (middle ear inflammation), choroidal plexus (meningitis), and the base of the hair shaft (poliosis may be a very common sign). The dysacusis may be manifest by tingling or deafness. Alopecia areata with poliosis and vitiligo, often the hallmarks of this disease, are common depigmented findings. Late findings of central nervous system vasculitis may include coma, paresis, disorientation, psychosis, and other underlying signs that may be diagnosed by abnormal electroencephalograms.

Aside from the anterior segment ocular disease appearing as a typical granulomatous iridocyclitis and vitritis, diffuse choroiditis with serous detachments of the retina is a common form of the disease and may occur in the absence of anterior segment inflammation (Harada's syndrome). The foci of choroiditis tend to include vasculitis in a focal fashion as well as the overall serous detachment of the retina as a late consequence of the blood vessel inflammation. Typical ocular signs of Vogt–Koyanagi–Harada disease such as iridocyclitis, pigment mottling

of the retinal pigment epithelium where previous serous detachment has occurred, poliosis, and vitiligo around the eyes may occur in the absence of any systemic complaints.

Vogt–Koyanagi–Harada syndrome

Definition
- A systemic inflammation with vasculitis in the retina, exudative detachment of the retina with choroiditis, etc.

Presentation
- Iridocyclitis
- Choroiditis
- Exudative retinal detachment
- Retinal vasculitis
- Granulomatous
- Poliosis
- ? Vitiligo

Investigation
- Lumbar puncture during attacks
- Fluorescein angiogram
- Medical consultation
- Skin and hair follicles biopsy for absence of melanocytes
- HLA BW22J
- HLA LDWa (Japan)
- HLA GR4
- HLA DQw3 (The West)

Therapy
- Intensive local systemic steroids
- Periocular steroids
- Low-dose local or systemic steroids in chronic cases
- Immunosuppressive agents (chlorambucil)
- Cyclosporin

Complications
- Cataract
- Glaucoma
- Optic nerve dysfunction
- Retinal vasculitis
- Retinal necrosis
- Phthisis

Prognosis
- Mixed, depending on the character of the case
- Its chronicity in particular is related to inflammatory activity
- Cataract surgery well tolerated
- All surgery poorly tolerated in chronically active cases

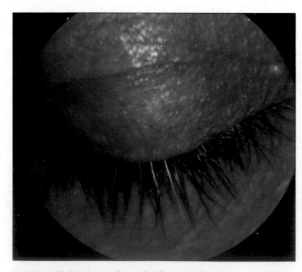

8.13 Whitening of eyelashes (poliosis) in a patient with Vogt–Koyanagi–Harada-type vitiligo change.

Table 8.2 Vogt–Koyanagi–Harada syndrome.

The disease appears to have a predilection for the more pigmented races, especially orientals. In Japan, Vogt–Koyanagi–Harada disease and Behçet's disease account for 25% of all cases of uveitis seen. The Harada's variety of Vogt–Koyanagi–Harada, in which only serous detachment of the retina occurs as an inflammatory manifestation in the absence of anterior inflammation, appears to be more common in Spanish-speaking people.

Fluorescein angiography of Vogt–Koyanagi–Harada disease is highly characteristic and may be very helpful in establishing the diagnosis. Choroiditis appears to block the vessels early, causing late leakage as in any typical vasculitis, and there is usually a marked accumulation of fluid in the subretinal space when serous detachments of the retina are occurring. The mottling of the retinal pigment epithelium, which is so typical after serous detachments, appears as a blocked hypofluorescence on fluorescein angiography.

All the clinical signs of Vogt–Koyanagi–Harada disease are similar to sympathetic ophthalmia, including

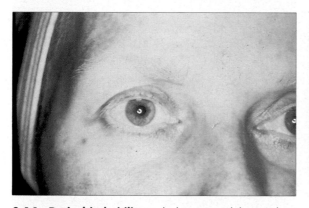

8.14 Periorbital vitiligo, which was so subtle as to be disguised completely by the patient's makeup. Only when it was requested that the makeup be removed did the facial vitiligo help to suggest the systemic and ocular diagnosis of Vogt–Koyanagi–Harada disease.

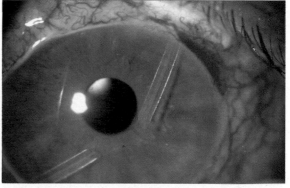

8.15 Double Moltino implant to control uveitic glaucoma in this patient with profound and unremitting iridocyclitis in Vogt–Koyanagi–Harada disease.

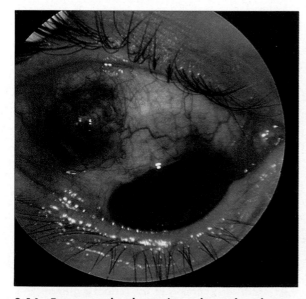

8.16 Extreme scleral ectasia and uveal prolapse in patient with vitiligo, poliosis, and panuveitis due to Vogt–Koyanagi–Harada disease.

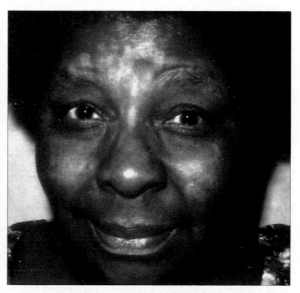

8.17 Marked obvious facial vitiligo in an African–American patient who has American–Indian heritage (Cherokee).

the vitiligo, poliosis, alopecia, and dysacusis. Sympathetic ophthalmia is also a granulomatous panuveitis that may occur as early as 2–4 weeks after a penetrating or very profound blunt injury to an eye in which uveal pigment is disturbed. It may occur up to 20 years after such an injury. There is a profound iridocyclitis and vitritis, and disseminated yellow-white nodules may be seen in the fundus (Dalen–Fuchs).

These nodules are inflammations in the retinal pigment epithelium itself where the pigment is phago-cytosed by epithelioid cells. In the pre-steroidal era useful vision was only achieved in 50% of eyes with sympathetic ophthalmia, but now more than 90% can be saved with combinations of steroidal and non-steroidal anti-inflammatory agents.

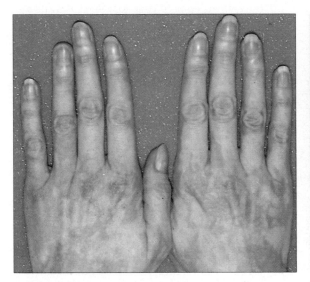

8.18 Vitiligo changes on the hands of a French patient with Vogt–Koyanagi–Harada disease.

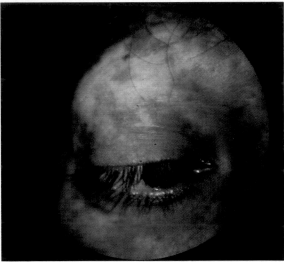

8.19 Marked and progressive vitiligo in a patient with an extreme iridocyclitis with Vogt–Koyanagi–Harada disease.

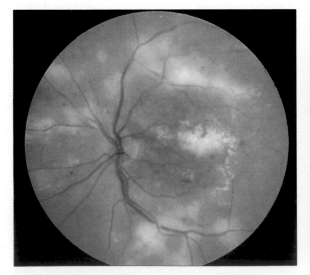

8.20 Marked exudative retinal detachment in a patient with Vogt–Koyanagi–Harada disease. Note the yellow exudative foci that are interspersed among the serous changes elevating the sensory retina.

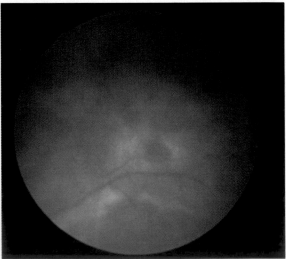

8.21 Marked scarring of the retinal pigment epithelium with fibrosis in a patient who has had recurrent exudative retinal detachment in Vogt–Koyanagi–Harada disease.

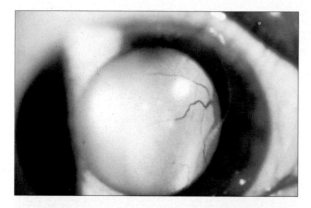

8.22 Extremely elevated yellow-coloured exudative retinal detachment noted at the slit lamp in a patient with Vogt–Koyanagi–Harada disease. Often, these exudative detachments can be so profound that they can elevate as high as the posterior lens capsule, as noted in this patient.

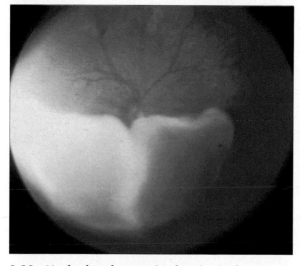

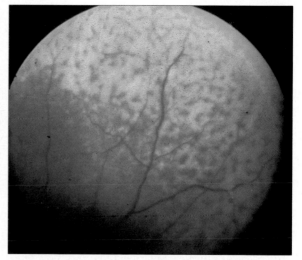

8.23 Marked and extensive hemiretinal exudative detachment in a patient with Vogt–Koyanagi–Harada disease.

8.24 Resolved recurrent exudative detachments in a patient with Vogt–Koyanagi–Harada disease showing the marked stippling hypertrophy and hypotrophy changes in the retinal pigment epithelium.

8.25 Patient with Vogt–Koyanagi–Harada disease after absorption of exudative retinal detachment. Note the fibrosis and scarring in the retinal pigment epithelium and the marked fibrosis leading to irretrievably decreased vision in this patient.

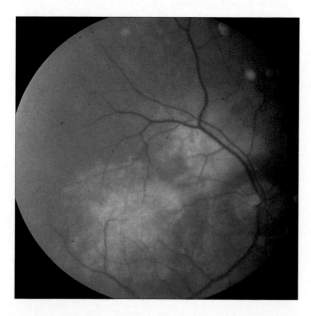

SARCOIDOSIS

Sarcoidosis (**8.26–8.37, Table 8.3**) is a multisystem disease whose histological hallmark is a noncaseating granuloma. Vasculitis and, more specifically, phlebitis are common accompaniments to the histological features of this disorder. Sarcoidosis accounts for 3–10% of all cases of uveitis and 25–50% of patients with systemic sarcoidosis develop uveal inflammation. The most common manifestation is iridocyclitis, but many different intraocular and extraocular structures may be involved.

Sarcoidosis is seen most commonly in Scandinavia and along the Atlantic Gulf coasts of the USA. In the USA it occurs 10 times more frequently in African–American patients than in Whites, with women outnumbering men 2:1. HLA B8 has been reported to occur more often in patients with sarcoid than in the general population. Although sarcoidosis has been reported in children and the elderly, it is most likely to occur in young and middle-aged patients.

For the majority of patients, ocular disease remains active for only several years, while less than 10% develop a chronic form of the disease for longer.

Systemic sarcoidosis usually involves the parenchyma of the lungs in 80% of patients. Hilar adenopathy involving the large lymph nodes draining the lungs may be seen in over 75% of patients, many of whom will be asymptomatic.

A gallium scan of the head and thorax will often demonstrate enlarged glandular tissue in the lacrimal area as well as in the salivary glands, and the adenopathy of the hilar region. Angiotensin-converting enzyme (ACE) should be obtained, but may be positive in the presence of other granulomatous diseases.

Sarcoidosis

Definition
- Granulomatous inflammation

Presentation
- Variable (great mimicker): iritis, vasculitis, granulomata
- Granulomatous

Investigation
- Chest radiograph
- Skin test (anergy to tuberculin, mumps, others)
- Conjunctival biopsy
- Erythrocyte sedimentation rate
- Consultation
- Angiotensin-converting enzyme (ACE)
- Serum lysozyme
- Gallium scan
- Serum proteins
- Serum and urinary calcium, phosphorus
- Radiography of hands, feet
- Kveim test

Therapy
- Local steroids
- Periocular steroids
- Treat recurrent iridocyclitis
- Treat chronic iridocyclitis
- Treat active choroiditis lesions with systemic steroids covered by antituberculous therapy (e.g. INH)

Prognosis
- Variable

Table 8.3 Sarcoidosis.

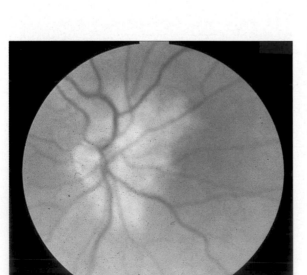

8.26 A 24-year-old white female presenting with optic nerve granuloma in acute sarcoidosis.

Skin manifestations of sarcoidosis are seen in approximately one-third of patients, while hepatomegaly will occur in only 15%. The eyelids and the conjunctivae should be carefully scanned with double eversion of the lids for sarcoid nodules, which may be of great benefit in yielding the histological hallmark of noncaseating granuloma. However, blind biopsy of the conjunctiva is considered fruitless.

A severe recurrent iridocyclitis occurs most frequently. Choroiditis and retinal vasculitis are often present and almost exclusively manifest as periphlebitis. The iridocyclitis is often characterized by large mutton-fat granulomatous keratic precipitates, dense posterior synechiae, peripheral anterior synechiae, and marked cell and flare in the anterior chamber.

The complications may be acute or chronic secondary glaucoma, band keratopathy, cataract, or granulomatous nodules on the iris surface, at the pupillary margin, in the stroma, and in the angle (Busacca, Koeppe, Berlin's nodules, respectively). Characteristically, many of these iris nodules become vascularized.

Sarcoidosis may manifest itself in the posterior segment of the eye, but not unless it is accompanied by anterior segment inflammation. Round yellow–grey lesions found in the choroid resolve, usually leaving a choroidal scar. When the retina itself is involved, there are usually exudates around the retinal vessels, predominantly on the venular side, described as 'candle wax drippings.' Snowball opacities in the vitreous cavity are usual and may be confused with those found in pars planitis. The optic nerve may be involved with a granuloma, causing resultant visual field defects in the central vision. Cystoid macular oedema may be a complication of the inflammation due to chronic phlebitis of the posterior segment of the eye.

Noncaseating epithelioid cell tubercle is the characteristic histological hallmark of sarcoidosis. The epithelioid cells probably derive from macrophages and often contain intermingled lymphocytes and multinucleated giant cells of the Langerhans type. Schaumann's bodies are characteristic inclusions found in the cytoplasm of the giant cells. The necrosis that is usually associated with tuberculosis is not found in sarcoidosis.

Infiltration of the glandular tissue of the lacrimal gland may produce a non-painful firm swelling in the supratemporal quadrant of the orbit and is be a common finding in patients with generalized systemic sarcoidosis. Other types of extraocular involvement include keratitis sicca and nodular infiltrations in both the bulbar and palpebral conjunctiva, which when recognized may offer a high percentage yield for diagnostic biopsy.

Corneal involvement in sarcoidosis is usually secondary to attendant hypercalcemia, and band keratopathy may sometimes be seen, as it is with an end-stage uveitis and glaucoma.

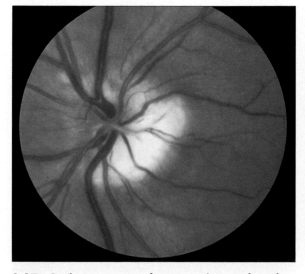

8.27 Optic nerve granuloma causing profound visual loss in young African–American patient. (Courtesy of Jonathan Belmont, MD.)

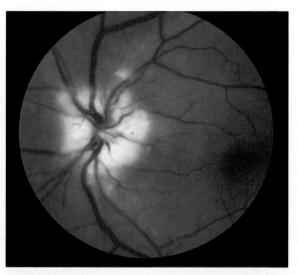

8.28 Fellow eye showing similar optic nerve granuloma with much more fluffy exudative material in an overlying parenchymal tissue of the optic nerve itself. (Courtesy of Jonathan Belmont, MD.)

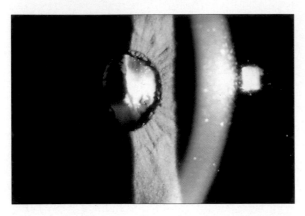

8.29 Synechiae and Koeppe nodule formation as well as fibrosis on the anterior lens capsule and profound iridocyclitis along with multiple keratic precipitates in a patient with acute sarcoid iridocyclitis.

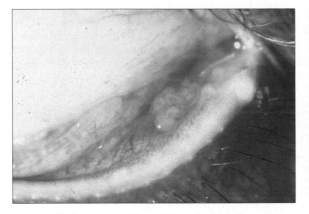

8.30 Obvious sarcoid nodule in the epibulbar region of the conjunctiva.

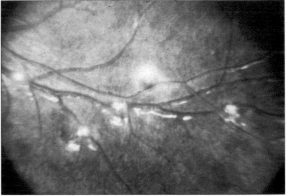

8.31 Exquisitely focal localized periphlebitis in a young African–American patient with sarcoidosis.

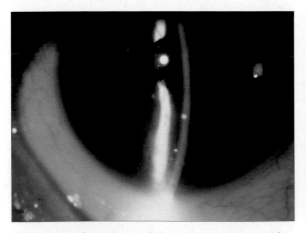

8.32 Large keratic precipitates in a patient with sarcoid iridocyclitis suggestive of its granulomatous histological nature.

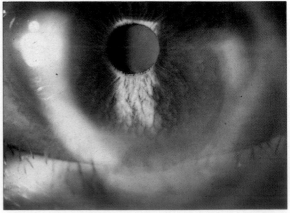

8.33 Marked demonstration of Busacca nodules in the iris of a patient with sarcoid uveitis.

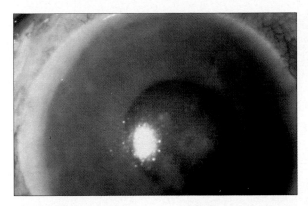

8.34 Large synechiae in a patient with sarcoid iridocyclitis.

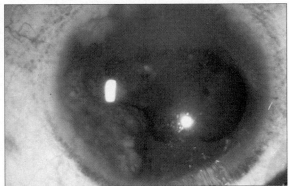

8.35 Giant iris granuloma distorting pupil in a patient with sarcoid iridocyclitis. (Courtesy of Jonathan Belmont, MD.)

8.36 Chest radiograph of a 24-year-old patient with systemic sarcoidosis demonstrating marked hilar adenopathy.

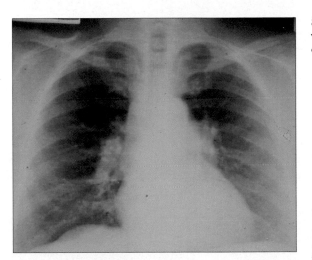

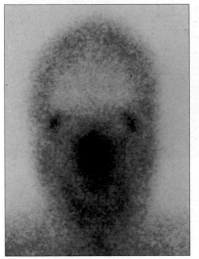

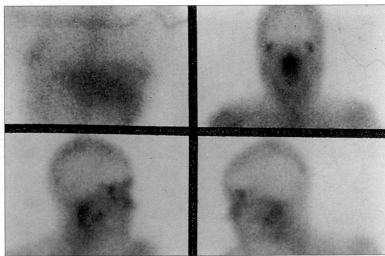

8.37a Gallium scan of head and neck showing sarcoid involvement of nasopharynx, and lacrimal and submandibular glands.

8.37b Montage of several views of gallium scan showing sarcoid uptake of the gallium in glandular tissue.

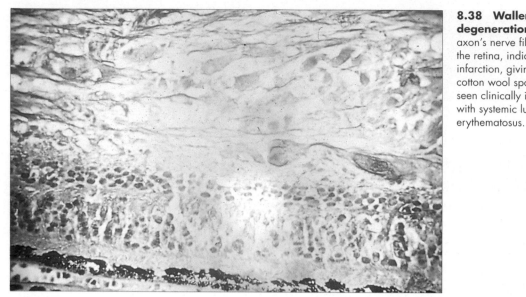

8.38 Wallerian degeneration of the axon's nerve fibre layer of the retina, indicative of infarction, giving rise to the cotton wool spots, which are seen clinically in the patient with systemic lupus erythematosus.

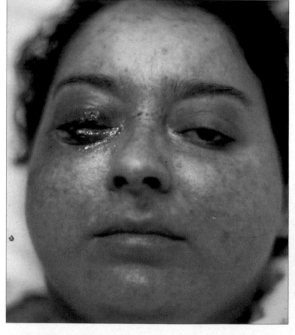

8.39 This patient with Cushingoid changes in the face from exogenous steroid administration for lupus erythematosus, had gangrene of the eyelid, which eventually sloughed just before the patient's death.

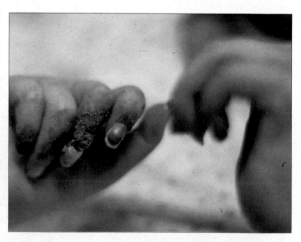

8.40 Fingertips of a patient with Raynaud's phenomena from systemic lupus erythematosus. Note the marked ischaemic changes in the very distal ends of the fingers and fingernails.

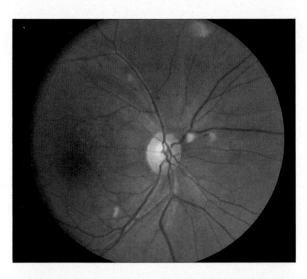

8.41 Marked vascular sheathing in a 32-year-old African–American female with the vasculitic changes of systemic lupus erythematosus.

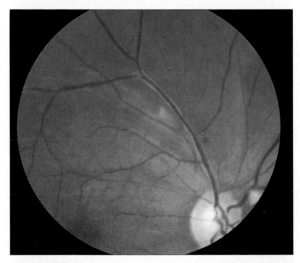

8.42 Fellow eye, same patient, showing vascular sheathing.

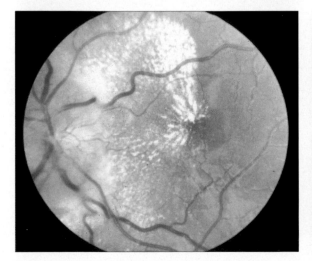

8.43 A 12-year-old white female showing hypertensive changes in the retina with macular scar formation and infarction of the nerve fibre layer.

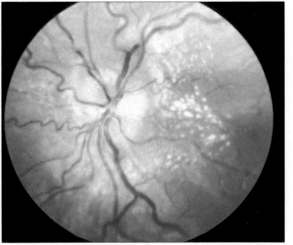

8.44 Fellow eye, same 12-year-old patient, showing marked hypertensive changes.

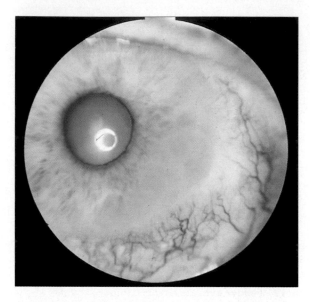

8.45 Ischaemic peripheral corneal melt in a patient with Wegener's granulomatosis.

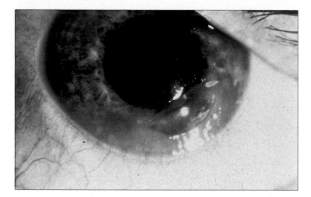

8.46 Marked ischaemia infratemporally on the sclera in a patient with contiguous corneal melt from Wegener's granulomatosis.

9.
Dermatological Disorders

Certain dermatological disorders are known to have ophthalmic manifestations, especially cicatricial pemphigoid.

CICATRICIAL PEMPHIGOID

Cicatricial pemphigoid demonstrates symblepharon formation, due to subepithelial fibrosis of the conjunctiva, usually involving the inferior fornix first with consequent corneal and conjunctival changes. Decreased vision is due to the corneal opacification resulting from exposure and irritation from inturned eyelashes. IgG bound to the conjunctival epithelial basal membrane is seen on direct immuno-fluorescence.

EPIDERMOLYSIS BULLOSA

Epidermolysis bullosa is a more broad-spectrum disease, which is characterised by skin fragility and blister formation, usually in response to some type of trauma. Some forms of the disease cause only minimal disability while others can be extremely disfiguring. The ocular manifestations usually include infiltrates and cystic lesions at the epithelial basement cell layer with blood formation in the corneal epithelium and a refractory blepharoconjunctivitis.

ERYTHEMA MULTIFORME OR STEVENS–JOHNSON SYNDROME

The most characteristic and severe dermatological syndrome of this group is erythema multiforme or Stevens–Johnson syndrome (**9.1**), which affects the mucous membranes including the conjunctiva. It is usually accompanied by fever and constitutional signs secondary to a vasculitis in the kidneys, heart, gastrointestinal tract, and central nervous system, and can be a life-threatening disease. A perivasculitis of the superficial dermal vessels occurs in which a mononuclear cell population is predominant. IgM and complement C3 are found in the walls of the skin vessels in the earliest phases of this disease.

A large percentage of cases occur 1–3 weeks after episodes of recurrent herpes simplex genitalis. The sulphonamides and other drugs, as well as a *Mycoplasma pneumoniae* infection, are known to be other causes of this very severe ocular and cutaneous disease.

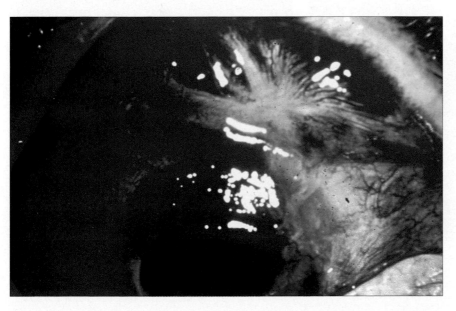

9.1 Epithelial cornification of cornea and conjunctiva with symblepharon formation in this elderly patient with Stevens–Johnson syndrome.

The conjunctival inflammation and scarring can be devastating with consequent tear insufficiency, conjunctival epithelial metaplasia, trichiasis, distichiasis, corneal ulceration, and corneal neovascularization.

Therapy for these manifestations is indicated to reduce the severity of epithelial scarring. If recurrent herpes simplex is the suspected aetiology, long-term suppressive doses of acyclovir may be necessary.

PEMPHIGUS

Pemphigus is a chronic bullous skin and mucous membrane disease that affects men and women who are usually in their fifth and sixth decades, and is described as thin flaccid bullae on normal-looking skin. While the fluid inside the bullae may be clear at first, it may later become haemorrhagic or seropurulent. These bullae rupture spontaneously with slight pressure or rubbing and become painful, with raw oozing erosions that bleed and are difficult to heal. The ocular involvement in pemphigus occurs in the conjunctiva and eyelids with hyperaemia, oedema, and trichiasis, and secondary infection due to crusting lesions in and around the eyelids.

JUVENILE XANTHOGRANULOMA

Juvenile xanthogranuloma is a benign histiocytic inflammatory disorder that affects mainly infants and small children. The skin and the eye are the two most common sites of involvement and usually there is spontaneous regression and disappearance of the lesions within 3 months to 6 years. The patient's general health is seldom impaired. The lesions are variable, elevated, and usually palpable. Histologically, there are nodular histiocytic proliferations in the subepidermal location.

The ocular manifestations, usually bilateral, include a mass in the iris, and less likely, the posterior choroid or retina. These may bleed spontaneously, and it is said that juvenile xanthogranuloma is a leading cause for spontaneous hyphaema in a youngster. Usually spontaneous hyperaemia or corneal oedema are present. Iridocyclitis has been reported.

PSEUDOXANTHOMA ELASTICUM

Pseudoxanthoma elasticum (PXE) (**9.2–9.15**) is a systemic disease in which the primary defect appears to be the production of elastin fibres with secondary calcification. Manifestations of the disease are seen in the skin, cardiovascular and pulmonary systems, and the eyes.

The systemic manifestations include the peau d'orange plaques in the skin, which are yellowish and xanthomatous and usually occur in areas of skin folds in the genital, popliteal and periumbilical regions, as well as the neck and underarms. The skin may feel velvety and thickened or atrophic, and usually has the appearance of a 'plucked chicken.' In some

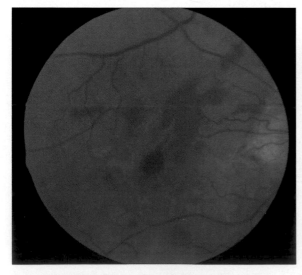

9.2 A fundal picture of angioid streaks with attendant haemorrhage in the retina, secondary to choroidal rupture and subretinal neovascularization.

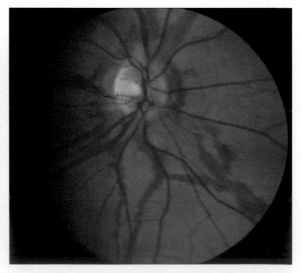

9.3 Marked demonstration of peripapillary streaking from angioid streaks, which represent weakness and rupture in Bruch's membrane. Note how these streaks circumvent the optic papilla and then radiate out from it.

areas, the affected skin appears wrinkled and redundant.

In the eyes, angioid streaks are the hallmark. These angioid streaks, which are bilateral and asymmetrical, are a clinical manifestation of breaks in Bruch's membrane at the choroidal–retinal junction. They usually form an incomplete ring around the optic nerve head and radiate toward the equator. As they represent a break in Bruch's membrane, they may result in choroidal neovascularization and may cause subretinal haemorrhage, especially in the macula. They need to be listed in the differential diagnosis of macular haemorrhage in young patients as distinct from macular degeneration or histoplasmosis.

Histopathologically, basophilia and calcification of Bruch's membrane corresponds to the clinical location of the angioid streaks. Hyperplastic or degenerative changes occur in the retinal pigment epithelium, and haemorrhagic detachment of the retinal pigment is noted with fibrovascular ingrowth.

The visual loss in PXE is directly related to the complications of macular haemorrhage and scarring. Less significant changes of PXE include a diffuse mottling of the retinal pigment epithelium or peau d'orange in the retina, which is akin to the skin changes, and appears as irregularly shaped, punched out lesions in the periphery alternating with dark pigment and light orange colour.

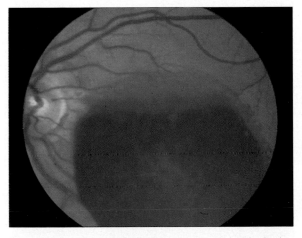

9.4 Subhyaloid haemorrhage in a patient who had a choroidal rupture from angioid streaks. Note how subtle the changes are around the optic nerve head and, in fact, these were indiscernible clinically.

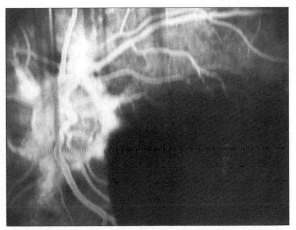

9.5 Fluorescein angiogram of the patient in 9.4 demonstrating the angioid streaks adjacent to the subhyaloid haemorrhage, which is obscuring the underlying choroidal fluorescence. Note how much more obvious these streaks are with angiographic demonstration as opposed to the clinical photography.

9.6 Angioid streak pattern of choroidal rupture, which is more obvious, radiating out supratemporally from the optic papilla.

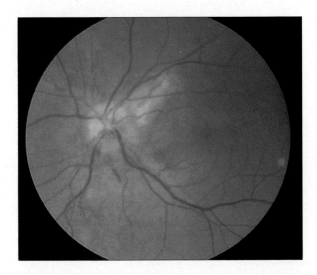

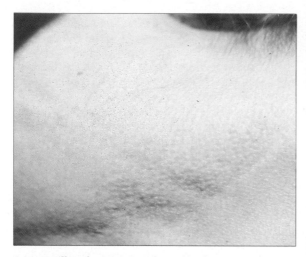

9.7 Axilla of patient with angioid streaks and pseudoxanthoma elasticum. Note the irregular and roughened epidermal surface.

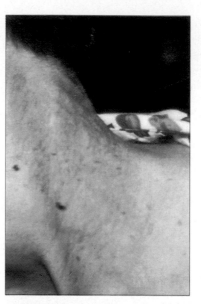

9.8 Neck of patient with pseudoxanthoma elasticum. Note the subtle colour change to the thickened rough skin, which is likened to a 'plucked chicken.'

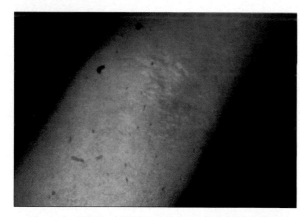

9.9 Antecubital region of arm of a patient with pseudoxanthoma elasticum.

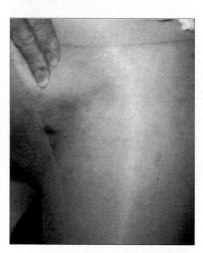

9.10 Note the inguinal streaks of roughened hyperpigmented epidermal change in this area, which is similar to that found in other skin areas where there are folds (i.e. behind the knees, the antecubital area, and the neck).

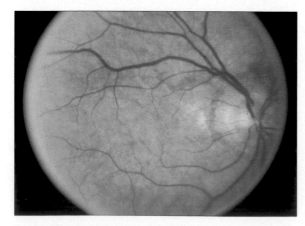

9.11 The typical peau d'orange hypopigmented changes in the retina typical of angioid streaks. Note the angioid streaks radiating superiorly off the optic nerve head.

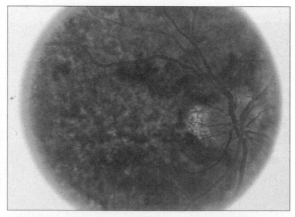

9.12 Fluorescein angiogram of the patient in 9.11 highlighting the peau d'orange changes in the retinal pigment epithelium as well as emphasizing the angioid streaks radiating superiorly off the optic nerve head.

Angioid streaks may also be seen in sickle cell anaemia, Paget's disease, familial hyperphosphataemia, metastatic calcification of the choroid in young females, idiopathic thrombocytopenic purpura, Ehlers–Danlos syndrome and lead poisoning. Any patient noted to have angioid streaks and/or PXE should be consulted by the internal medicine specialist for the presence of changes that may occur concurrently or later in the cardiovascular or pulmonary system and lead to unexpected morbidity and death in these patients.

It must be remembered that other systemic disorders may be associated with angioid streaks other than PXE (Grönblad–Strandberg syndrome). These would include Ehlers–Danlos syndrome of fibrodysplasia hyperelastica, senile elastosis, Paget's disease of the bone (osteitis deformans), chronic congenital idiopathic hyperphosphataemia (a juvenile form of Paget's disease), calcinosis, acromegaly, sickle cell haemoglobinopathy, thalassemia acanthocytosis, and hereditary spherocytosis.

PSORIASIS

Psoriasis is a common skin disorder that affects 2% of the population of the United States. It occurs at any age, but usually begins in older childhood or young adulthood. The characteristic skin lesions are large, well-defined, multiple pink–red patches covered by white–silver scales.

The ocular manifestations can take several forms. Psoriatic patches may involve the lids (**9.16**) and can even extend onto the conjunctiva. Chronic blephari-

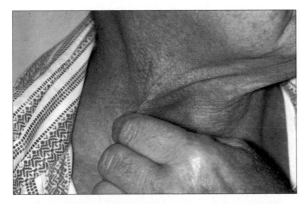

9.13 Pinching of the epidermal areas on the neck in pseudoxanthoma elasticum.

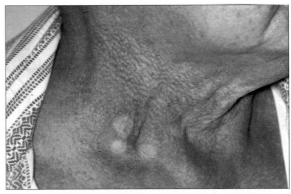

9.14 Notice how the elasticity changes will maintain the 'pinch' and are highlighted by the easily ischaemic manifestations around it.

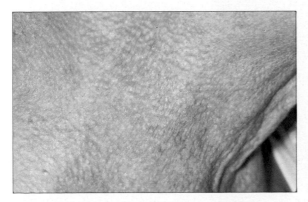

9.15 Higher magnification of the 'plucked chicken' appearance of the neck in a patient with pseudoxanthoma elasticum and angioid streaks.

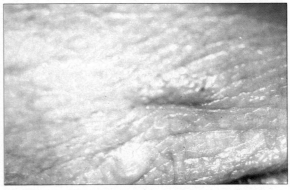

9.16 Crusting white eyelid lesion of psoriasis.

127

tis and lash loss occur frequently in this form. Nonspecific conjunctivitis, cicatricial conjunctival changes, symblepharon, trichiasis, and dry eye may occur. Peripheral corneal opacities, ulcer or keratopathy with stromal melting, and forms of keratitis resembling rosacea may also be present. The incidence of cataract does not increase in psoriatic patients. Uveitis may occur as a complication of psoriasis and cause visual loss, but is infrequent.

ACNE ROSACEA

Acne rosacea is characterized by erythema telangiectasis of the sun-exposed areas of the malar region of the face and upper chest. The dermatological lesions are characterized by erythema, telangiectasis, papules, pustules, sebaceous gland hypertrophy, and flush over the face and chest, usually the malar regions and the eyelids (**9.17**).

Rosacea occurs most commonly in the age range of 20–60 years and is rare in children.

Ocular involvement occurs in more than 50% of patients, and includes chronic blepharitis, meibomianitis, chalazia, papillary conjunctivitis, episcleritis, and superficial punctate keratopathy, and in its most severe form, infiltrative and ulcerative keratopathy with infected ulceration. Vascularization of the peripheral cornea may occur with subepithelial infiltrates. Usually these are confined to the inferior two-thirds of the cornea, but ultimately may become ulcerated and vascularized through the entire cornea. It is reported that one-third of patients with rosacea who are referred to an ophthalmologist have keratitis sicca.

ATOPY

All forms of atopy may occur in the ophthalmology population, demonstrating a chronic pruritic erythematous inflammation of the skin in conjunction with a variety of ocular manifestations, including dermatitis of the lids, loss of the lateral portions of the eyebrows secondary to rubbing, prominent folds of the lower lids beginning at the inner canthi, as well as diffuse papillary hypertrophy and a hyperaemic oedematous conjunctiva. Clear epithelial inclusion cysts and Trantas' dots are occasionally present along with symblepharon, conjunctival distortion, and trichiasis. Corneal involvement includes pannus, epithelial keratitis, and stromal haze. Ulcerations and vascularization are also reported in the cornea. The relationship between atopy and keratoconus remains controversial, but cataracts are found in up to 25% of patients with atopic dermatitis of the anterior subcapsular types or posterior subcapsular type.

DERMATOLOGICAL MANIFESTATIONS OF OTHER SYSTEMIC DISEASES

Dermatological manifestations of other systemic diseases shown in this chapter have detailed descriptions in other chapters include sarcoidosis (**9.18–9.20**), discoid lupus (**9.21**), skin manifestations of herpes zoster ophthalmicus (note in **9.22** that the nasociliary division of V is infected, clearly implicating corneal involvement in this patient), molluscum contagiosum (**9.23 and 9.24**), vaccinia involving the lids (**9.25 and 9.26**), dermatomyositis (**9.27**), and lepromatous skin changes (**9.28 and 9.29**).

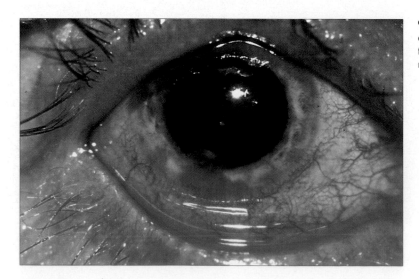

9.17 Violaceous eyelid margins as well as malar and palpebral telangiectasia in a patient with acne rosacea.

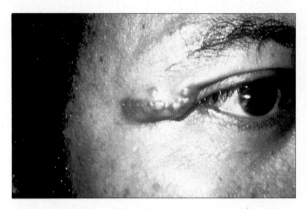

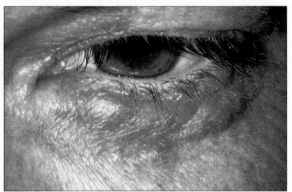

9.18 Lateral canthus of a patient with systemic sarcoidosis demonstrating the classical thickened, rubbery, epidermal and dermal lesion of lupus pernio indicative of this granulomatous disease.

9.19 Lower lid demonstrating thickening erythema and rubbery appearance of sarcoid nodules in a patient with systemic sarcoidosis.

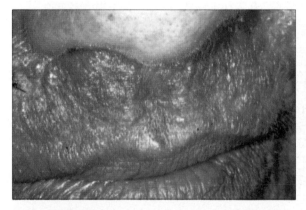

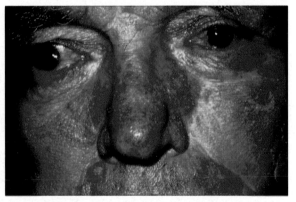

9.20 Thickened, red elevated area of epidermal nodulation indicative of lupus pernio in a patient with systemic sarcoidosis.

9.21 Extensive discoid lupus changes in the skin over nose, forehead, and malar eminence in this patient as well as conjunctival and episcleral involvement.

9.22 Classic hemifacial dermatome distribution of herpes zoster ophthalmicus. Note the lesion on the tip of the nose indicative of nasociliary involvement, which implies ocular infection.

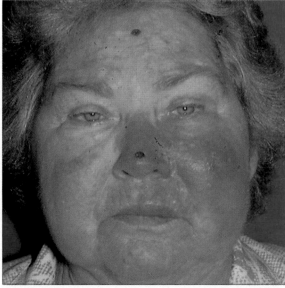

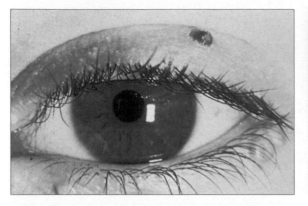

9.23 Elevated erythematous lesion of molluscum contagiosum in the eyelid of a 12-year-old child.

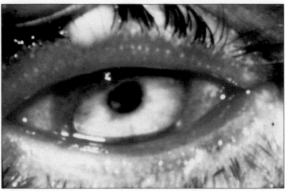

9.24 Palpebral lesions of molluscum contagiosum.

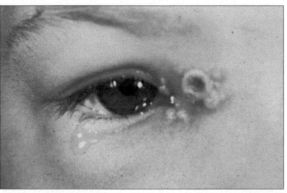

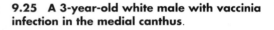

9.25 A 3-year-old white male with vaccinia infection in the medial canthus.

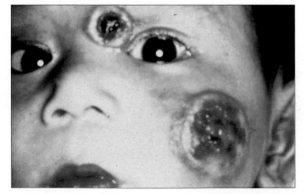

9.26 A 4-year-old with extensive lesions of vaccinia on the medial and upper canthus and the lateral malar region.

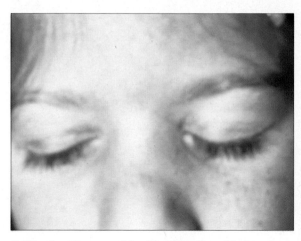

9.27 An 11-year-old white female with the violaceous hue on the upper lids in dermato-myositis.

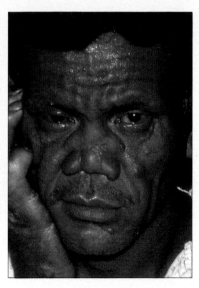

9.28 The typical leonine facies of a patient with lepromatous leprosy. Note that the distal digit of the little finger on the right hand is missing due to involvement in the finger.

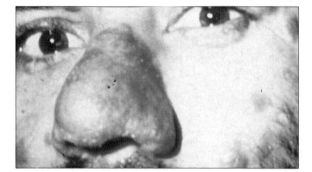

9.29 Bulbus erythematous nose as well as facial skin lesions of lepromatous leprosy.

10.
Drug Toxicity

Drug toxicity (**Table 10.1**) is common in ophthalmology and is usually associated with prolonged use of topical ophthalmic medications. Often, it is initiated by the ophthalmologist's prescription, but frequently it is perpetuated by the patient and their overuse of eyedrops and ointment. The idea that 'if a little medication is good, a lot of medication is better,' is a concept that aggravates the situation.

Many commonly used ophthalmic medications are toxic when used in excessive amounts or for long periods of time. Patients often begin eyedrops for red eyes or irritation. Cosmetic concerns about red eyes are perhaps the most common reasons for excessive use of eyedrops. With persistent use, generally after 2 or 3 weeks, redness persists or becomes worse. This may cause the patient to use even more eyedrops or perhaps switch to a different eyedrop.

Multiple visits to ophthalmologists may lead to the acquisition of more prescription eyedrops. Sometimes several different kinds of eyedrops are used within the course of a day. This leads to persistent redness and a papillary reaction of the upper and lower tarsal conjunctiva (**10.1 and 10.2**). If the drug is continued, keratinization of the conjunctiva (**10.3**) or cicatrization of the conjunctiva (**10.4**) may occur. Epithelial defects of the inferior cornea and bulbar conjunctiva frequently occur. If exposure to the toxic drug continues, large epithelial defects may result (**10.5**). Drug toxicity may be a combination of

Drug toxicity
Definition
• Deleterious effect to the eye due to excessive or prolonged use of a topical or systemic medication
Presentation
• Conjunctivitis
• Keratitis
• Corneal epithelial defects
• Conjunctival scarring
• Corneal deposits
Investigation
• Meticulous history
• Involvement of inferior cornea and conjunctiva
• Improvement on discontinuing the drug
Therapy
• Discontinuation of the drug
• Tear substitution with unpreserved artificial tears and compresses
Complications
• Conjunctival scarring
• Corneal scarring
Prognosis
• Excellent

Table 10.1   Drug toxicity.

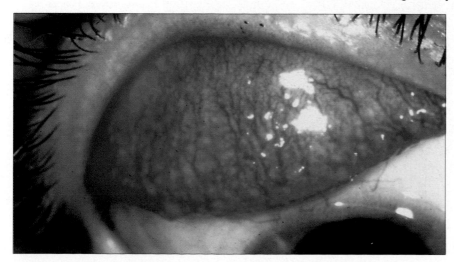

10.1 Papillary hypertrophy of the upper tarsal conjunctiva in a patient with toxicity to multiple topical drugs.

primary irritancy from the offending compound and contact allergy, a from of allergy mediated by lymphocytes rather than antibodies.

Patients with drug toxicity complain of a foreign body sensation, blurred vision, and extreme photophobia. Ther is usually a history of indiscriminate use of eyedrops for several weeks or months. Often the photophobia is out of proportion to the other symptoms. Patients suffering from drug toxicity are often so sensitive that the examining room lights are painful, so they insist on being in a darkened room. Obviously, this makes it difficult to examine their eyes with the slit-lamp microscope. There may also be a skin reaction involving the lower lid preferentially. There may be a breakdown of the skin of the eyelid, particularly at the lateral and medial canthus. There may be a variable amount of erythema and oedema. There may also be a mild, moderate or severe corneal involvement characterized by fluorescent staining, especially in the lower half of the cornea.

Sometimes a contact allergic reaction is superimposed on a toxic reaction. It may, in fact, be difficult to separate the toxic from the allergic component. Some drugs, such as neomycin and idoxuridine, are good contact sensitizers, but they also have inherent toxic properties. Preservatives such as thimesotal are

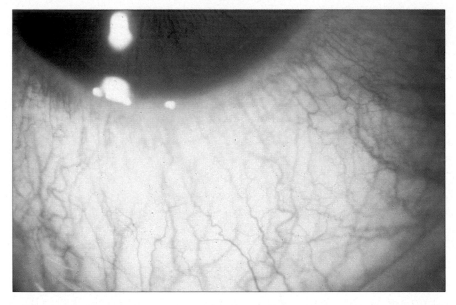

10.2 Allergic conjunctivitis with mild erythema and moderate chemosis.

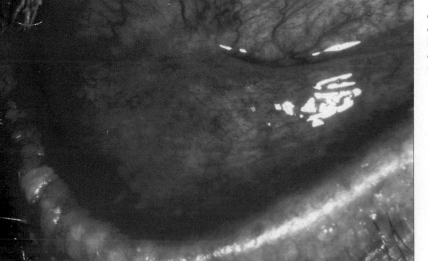

10.3 Keratinization and cicatrization of the conjunctiva, both on the bulbar palpebral conjunctiva, in a patient with topical drug toxicity.

also good contact sensitives, although they are less commonly found in ophthalmic preparations than in the past.

Fortunately, the treatment for drug toxicity is fairly simple. The toxic medication must be discontinued and an improvement is usually seen within a day of discontinuation. Depending upon how severe the toxicity is, it may take several days or even weeks for the toxic signs to resolve. Artificial tears, especially those without preservative, and either warm or cold compresses may be used in the interim.

Occasionally systemic drugs may be deposited in the eye. One of the most common is amiodarone, a cardiac drug, which is deposited in the cornea in a swirl-like pattern (cornea verticillata) (**10.6**). There is usually no reduction in vision and the corneal deposits are not an indication that the drug needs to be discontinued. Similar patterns of drug deposition can be seen with chloroquine, indomethacin, phenothiazine, suramin, and chlorpromazine.

Graft-versus-host disease may be seen 10–20 days after bone marrow implantation (**10.7**). It is characterized by fever, maculo-papular rash and severe dry eye. The rash may disappear or evolve into a chronic form of the disease.

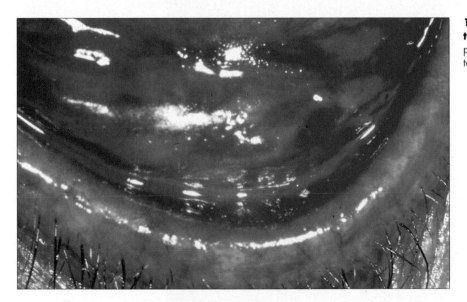

10.4 Cicatrization of the conjunctiva in a patient with a severe drug toxicity.

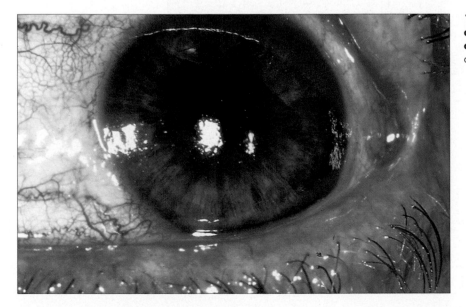

10.5 Epithelial disturbance of the cornea in a patient with a drug reaction.

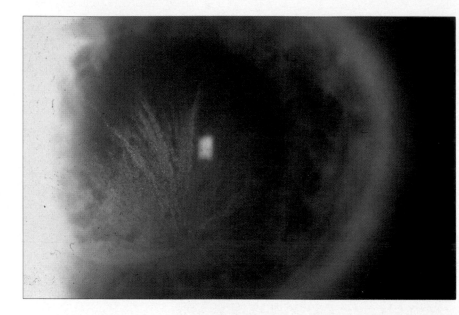

10.6 Amiodarone deposition in the cornea of a 63-year-old female patient.

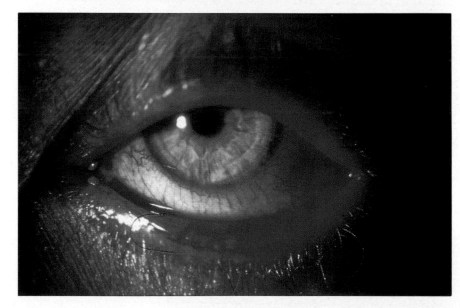

10.7 Graft-versus-host reaction with dryness and lid inflammation following bone marrow transplantation.

11.
Ophthalmological Recognition of Systemic Drug Abuse

One of the most pervasive problems facing our society today is drug abuse. Disgruntled segments of society are prone to the seduction of drugs and their mood-altering capabilities. The feelings of alienation, stress, grief, and depression can be and often are chemically alleviated.

Drugs of abuse can be 'snorted,' smoked, injected into the soft tissues ('skin popping', **11.1 and 11.2**), or injected directly into a vein ('mainlining', **11.3**). The most profound morbidity of drug abuse is associated with the intravenous injection of drugs. Desperate patients who run out of venous access sites may inject into surprising areas, such as soft tissues around the breast in women, or the dorsum of the penis. Short of venous access, some substance users will inject joint spaces and bursae at the joints, and even soft tissue spaces between fingers and toes. Skin tattoos may camouflage sclerosed or discolored skin at injection sites and may serve to alert the clinician to the patient's concealed substance abuse (**11.4 and 11.5**).

Complications of drug abuse include physical or chemical injury, and bacterial, fungal, protozoal, and viral infections.

The intravenous drug abuser is susceptible to a vast array of infections of all organ systems. Total disregard for aseptic technique, contaminated illicit drugs and diluting substances, sharing of injection

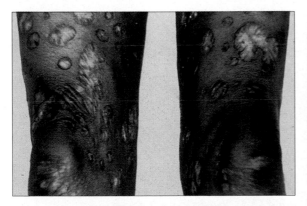

11.1 Legs of a patient with extensive scarring due to 'skin popping,' which is the subdermal method of substance injection used primarily when blood vessel access has run out.

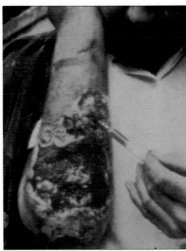

11.2 Graphic demonstration of desperation of patient who continues to 'skin pop' long after he has developed profound necrobiosis of the skin and an infection secondary to his injection routine.

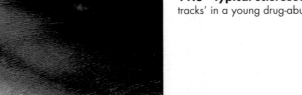

11.3 Typical sclerosed vessel, which belies 'needle tracks' in a young drug-abusing patient.

paraphernalia by several people, and the direct infusion of organisms into the blood and subcutaneous tissue are all responsible for these devastating complications of parenteral drug abuse.

Bacterial infections of the heart (endocarditis) or eye (endophthalmitis) in an otherwise healthy young person should suggest the possibility of parenteral drug abuse.

Fungi, most commonly *Candida* species, are responsible for endophthalmitis with a resultant high mortality rate among intravenous drug users. More than 20% of fungal endocarditis cases are associated with parenteral drug abuse.

Acquired immunodeficiency syndrome (AIDS) is the deadliest infectious complication of parenteral drug abuse. The use of intravenous drugs predisposes to AIDS through the transmission of the human immunodeficiency virus (HIV). Almost one in four patients with AIDS in the USA is a parenteral drug abuser. Studies in New York and other large eastern cities show that nearly 80% of intravenous drug abusers have antibody to the HIV. Male intravenous drug addicts frequently transmit the HIV to their female sexual consorts, and these women may transmit the infection to their children. In the future, many of the presently asymptomatic HIV-infected drug addicts and their sexual contacts will develop severe opportunistic infections and unusual neoplasms as a result of acquired immune deficiency.

OCULAR COMPLICATIONS OF DRUG ABUSE

The ocular complications of drug abuse (**Table 11.1**) include pharmacological effects, physiological manifestations, interpretational phenomena, and infectious diseases.

Systemic drug abuse

Definition
- Ocular signs that intravenous or subcutaneous particulate substances are injected and absorbed into vitreous, retina, choroid

Presentation
- Vitreous fluff balls
- Endophthalmitis
- Particulate retinal embolism
- Vitritis
- Usually in otherwise healthy young person
- Drug abuse usually denied initially

Investigation
- Ultrasound of globe
- Paracentesis of anterior/posterior chamber for bacteria, fungi
- Directed biopsy of vitreous for fungi

Therapy
- Specific treatment for fungal/bacterial aetiology

Complications
- Panuveitis
- Cataract
- Retinal detachment
- Glaucoma
- Phthisis and loss of eye
- Patient noncompliance
- Psychological problems

Prognosis
- Usually poor
- Good if *Candida* endophthalmitis diagnosed and treated early

Table 11.1   Systemic drug abuse

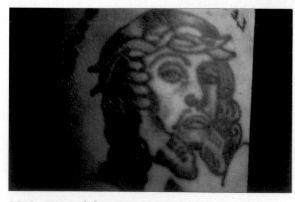

11.4   More elaborate tatoo in an intravenous drug abuser used to camouflage needle access routes, but also proclaims religious significance.

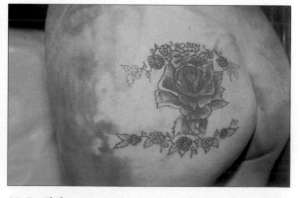

11.5   Elaborate tatoo on a young female patient who died of intravenous drug abuse.

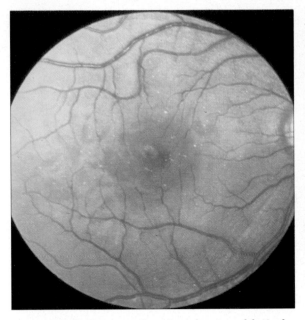

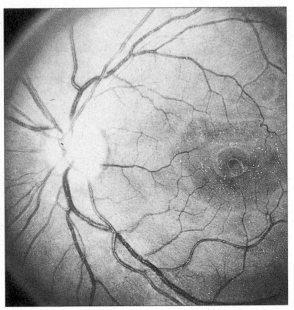

11.6 Small, discrete glistening shower of foci of injected particles in a patient with ritalin emboli from intravenous drug abuse.

11.7 Fluorescein angiogram of patient in 11.6 highlighting more extensively the shower of ritalin particles embolizing into retina.

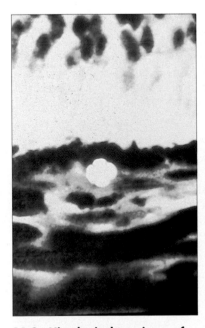

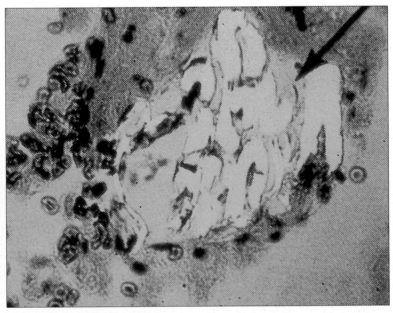

11.8 Histological specimen of retina demonstrating cotton embolism, which accompanied injection of intravenous material. Cotton strands often affect patients when used as an accompaniment to 'purify' the injected substance.

11.9 Cotton embolism in lung where it was strained out from its vascular injection.

OPIATES

The opiates have many physiological effects on the eye. The most prominent feature is a decrease in the size of the pupil by an unknown mechanism. Pupillary constriction can still be observed as a delayed effect in addicts who have not used narcotics recently. Other ocular side-effects of narcotics include ptosis, nystagmus, diplopia, and blurred vision.

MARIJUANA

Marijuana, the third most used recreational drug after alcohol and tobacco, is a mixture of leaves and flowers of the hemp plant, *Cannabis sativa*.

The ocular side-effects of marijuana include conjunctival hyperaemia, photophobia, diplopia, nystagmus, blepharospasms, ciliary injection of the globe, increased visibility of the corneal nerves, and decreased accommodation. Alteration of colour vision, including dichromatopsia, yellow vision, coloured flashing lights, and heightened colour perception has been reported.

The active ingredient in marijuana, delta-9-tetrahydrocannabinol (THC), decreases intraocular pressure by 25% after smoking or oral ingestion. THC has been proven to be an effective adjunctive drug for the treatment of glaucoma.

AMPHETAMINES OR STIMULANTS

Amphetamines or stimulants have multiple ocular side-effects including mydriasis, decreased accommodation and convergence, visual hallucinations, problems with colour vision, posterior subcapsular cataract formation, and decreased vision. In addition, mydriasis of the pupil can precipitate narrow angle glaucoma.

COCAINE

Cocaine dilates the pupil indirectly by preventing reuptake of norepinephrine. This mechanism is active only if sympathetic innervation is intact.

In high concentrations, cocaine causes cycloplegia with a dilated pupil. Cocaine also decreases accommodation and may lead to exophthalmos and retraction of the upper eyelid. Cocaine was one of the earliest analgesics for topical use in the eye, and when instilled locally has an anaesthetic effect that can produce corneal drying due to lack of blinking.

BARBITURATES

The ocular effects of barbiturates include ptosis, jerky pursuit movements of the eyes, random ocular movements, diplopia, decreased convergence, nystagmus, dyschromatopsia, yellow or green tinge to vision, visual hallucinations, retinal vasoconstriction, and subconjunctival haemorrhages secondary to drug-induced anaemia. Optic nerve disorders reportedly due to barbiturates include retrobulbar or optic neuritis, papilloedema, and optic atrophy.

NON-BARBITURATE DEPRESSANTS

Nonbarbiturate depressants, including methaqualone, have been associated with eyelid oedema, ptosis, nystagmus, diplopia, blurred vision, and visual hallucinations. An overdose of methaqualone has been reported to cause bilateral retinal haemorrhages that may clear completely in 6 weeks. In excessive doses, methaqualone can cause purpura and conjunctival haemorrhages. It is unclear whether this is secondary to an acute toxic effect of the drug, disseminated intravascular coagulopathy, or generalized hypoxia with increased capillary permeability and fragility.

HALLUCINOGENIC OR PSYCHEDELIC DRUGS

The hallucinogenic or psychedelic drugs have the ability to produce hallucinations and to separate the individual from reality and produce profound disturbances in cognition and perception. Changes in perception can be viewed as an ocular side-effect. Phencyclidine (PCP) has the reported side-effects of ptosis, paucity of spontaneous eye movements, and decreased corneal reflex. A particular array of ocular movement disorders has been associated with PCP as well as other hallucinogens. While primary gaze may be normal, patients show striking bursts of irregular jerky nystagmus occurring on either horizontal or vertical gaze, but most markedly on upward gaze. Prolonged visual perceptive disturbances in patients who have taken hallucinogenic drugs may go on for months. Hallucinogen abusers have also been reported to have flashback phenomena occurring months to years after usage of these drugs. Even after occasional use these flashbacks may be a driving or occupational hazard. Patients who abuse drugs of this category in particular are noted to 'sun gaze' or stare at the sun. This may cause a profound solar burn in the retina or the macula, irreversibly reducing vision.

CONGENITAL MALFORMATIONS ASSOCIATED WITH DRUGS OF ABUSE

Congenital malformations in newborns have been reported to be associated with many drugs of abuse.

Lysergic acid diethylamide (LSD) has been shown to cause chromosomal abnormalities *in vitro* and *in vivo*. Many infants have been born with brain and eye abnormalities to mothers who took large quantities of amphetamines, marijuana, and LSD. The most frequent eye abnormalities reportedly associated with these drugs have been atrophic optic nerves and bilateral cataract development. Additionally, unilateral coloboma of the iris, cataract formation, corneal opacification, and vascularization of intraocular tissues have all been reported in association with maternal drug abuse, but these conditions may also be observed in the general population due to spontaneous mutations.

FUNGAL ENDOPHTHALMITIS

Fungal endophthalmitis is the most serious and increasingly common ocular complication of intravenous drug abuse (**11.10**). The use of unsterile needles and syringes leads to the dissemination of a wide variety of organisms into the blood. Endophthalmitis

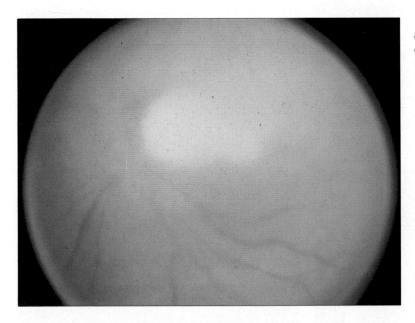

11.10 A 20-year-old male with classic picture of *Candida* endophthalmitis secondary to intravenous drug abuse.

may be secondary to infection with bacteria, fungi, or protozoans. The most common fungal agent is the *Candida* species. Most of these patients develop an anterior chamber inflammatory reaction and substantial vitreous clouding. Abscess formation on the retinal surface is a late potential consequence.

The most common clinical presentation of *Candida* endophthalmitis is a white fluffy ball of inflammation usually located in the vitreous, then extending onto the retina (**11.11–11.13**). It may later extend into all the ocular tissues.

The diagnosis of *Candida* endophthalmitis requires a high level of suspicion on the part of the physician. A thorough history focusing particularly on known risk factors should be sought. If the typical retinal or vitreous signs are present in a high-risk patient, a vitreous specimen is essential to make a definitive diagnosis. Anterior chamber paracentesis may yield organisms on culture, but usually a diagnostic vitrectomy is necessary. A diagnostic vitreous suction biopsy by needle aspiration may lead to retinal detachment and further ocular deterioration. Controlled cutting and sucking with a vitreous biopsy instrument is the safest means to obtain vitreous gel for examination and culture.

Candida endophthalmitis demonstrates either granulomatous inflammation or an acute suppurative reaction with necrosis histologically.

Most eyes have multiple lesions, generally measuring less than 1 mm in diameter, which are located in the posterior pole. The lesions are slightly elevated with a smooth surface and underlying deep pigmentation leading to a transillumination defect in the retinal pigment epithelium.

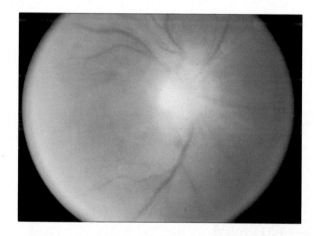

11.11 Another patient showing dense vitritis and puff ball overlying the optic papilla due to *Candida* endophthalmitis and drug abuse.

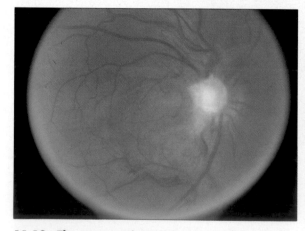

11.12 The same patient as in 11.11 after pars plana vitrectomy showing the resolution of the vitreous infiltration and the healing of the infection on the optic nerve head and adjacent retina.

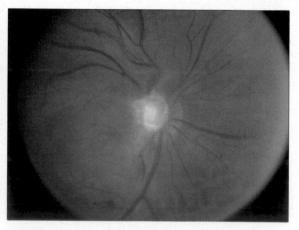

11.13 *Candida* endophthalmitis of patient in 11.11 medically resolved with resolution of normal and useful vision.

Aspergillus endophthalmitis is the second commonest fungus described in the PDAs (Parental Drug Abusers). This ubiquitous organism may be cultured from the normal human respiratory tract as well as from dust and air.

Aspergillus endophthalmitis has an exceptionally poor prognosis, and only four cases in the literature report saving the eye (**11.14–11.19**). Initial visual complaints include decreased visual acuity, pain, and conjunctival injection. Almost all cases have been unilateral. Anterior chamber reaction is seen along with keratic precipitates, conjunctival injection, and a profound vitreal and retinal infection.

Hyphaema, concomitant vitreous inflammation, and masses have been described. Retinal detachment and necrosis have also been described in many of these cases.

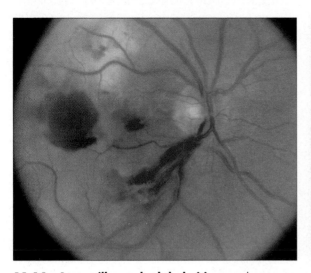

11.14 *Aspergillus* **endophthalmitis** secondary to intravenous drug abuse.

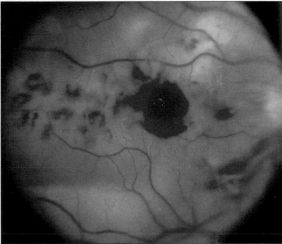

11.15 The same patient as in 11.14 showing meniscus of subretinal exudation as well as profound haemorrhagic and inflammatory change in the retina secondary to *Aspergillus* endophthalmitis in a 24-year-old white male drug abuser.

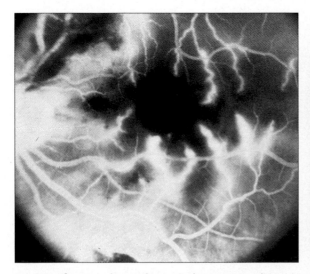

11.16 Fluorescein angiogram demonstrating the profound vasculitis accompanying this *Aspergillus* endophthalmitis.

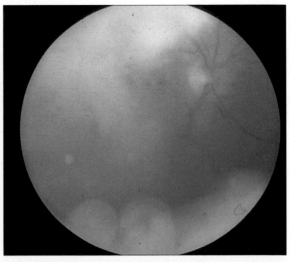

11.17 Another patient with *Aspergillus* endophthalmitis secondary to intravenous drug abuse where the vitreous is so cloudy from dense white exudation that very little of the retina can be visualized.

BACTERIAL ENDOPHTHALMITIS

Bacterial endophthalmitis as an ocular complication of drug abuse is reported much less often than mycotic endophthalmitis. Most reported cases have been associated with acute bacterial endocarditis, commonly with an organism of high pathogenicity. Staphylococcal species are the predominant organisms, accounting for 75% of reported cases. Diagnosis requires a high degree of suspicion on the part of the physician. Surgical confirmation is necessary because the antibiotics required have severe side-effects.

TALC RETINOPATHY

Talc retinopathy has been associated with the abuse of intravenous ritalin, heroin, methadone, cocaine, demerol, and talwin. Ritalin tablets contain talc (magnesium silicate) and cornstarch as fillers and binders and are meant for oral use. Only after prolonged intra-

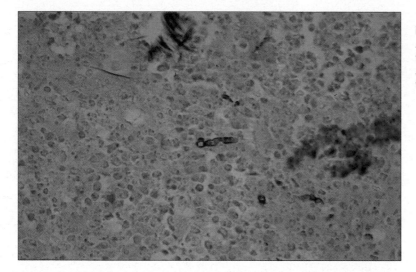

11.18 Histological section of rib in patient in 11.17 demonstrating *Aspergillus* osteomyelitis as a life-threatening accompaniment to his *Aspergillus* endophthalmitis secondary to his intravenous drug abuse.

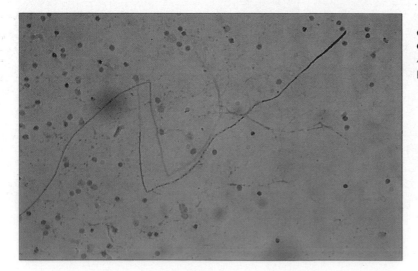

11.19 Histological demonstration of vitreous aspirate in a patient showing *Aspergillus* hyphae recovered at pars plana vitrectomy surgery.

venous drug abuse with resultant pulmonary hypertension, cor pulmonale, and pulmonary vascular collateral development do talc particles pass into the systemic circulation where they come to rest in end organs such as the eye. In the eye, most of these particles settle out in the posterior retinal and choroidal circulation due to the dense capillary network in this region.

Ophthalmoscopy reveals tiny, glistening, yellow crystals concentrated along the small arterioles of the perifoveal arcade and the posterior pole. Microaneurysmal dots, enlarged arterial segments, and venous loops may also be observed.

The talc or cornstarch emboli are found in the nerve fibre layer or choriocapillaris. Actual cotton emboli (from the 'filtering' of injected substances) may be found either clinically or histopathologically. Bilateral visual loss and irreversible macular ischaemia from talc emboli have been described in an intravenous ritalin abuser.

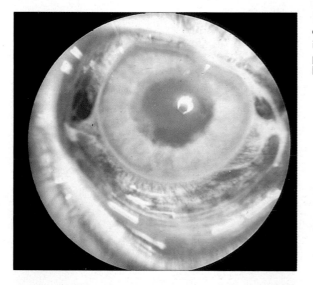

11.20 Acute haemorrhagic sclerosing of conjunctiva secondary to repeated amphotericin B injections, which are painful and vasoconstricting to the patient. Note that the circumpupillary vasculature has haemorrhaged with this series of injections.

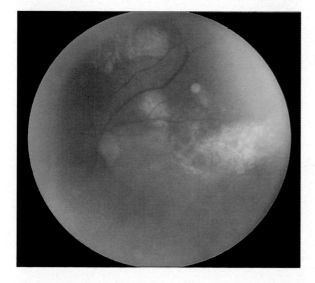

11.21 'Recovered' fundus view of patient in 11.10–11.13 demonstrating sclerosis of the retinal pigment epithelium and choroid, but with salvaged fovea, giving this patient 20/50 vision.

145

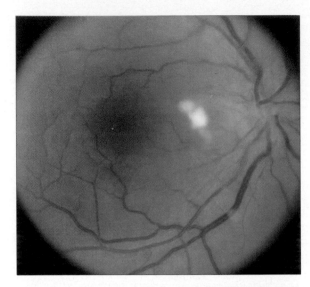

11.22 Acute glistening embolism from intravenous cocaine injection in a patient who suffered acute metamorphopsia and ocular migraine-type syndrome after injecting the substance at a party.

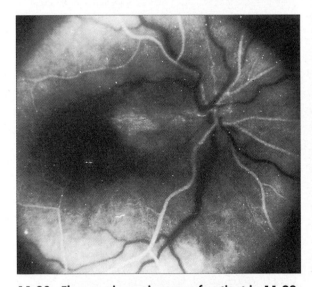

11.23 Fluorescein angiogram of patient in 11.22 showing the embolism as a very early stage of inflammation and particle in the papular–macular bundle in the right eye.

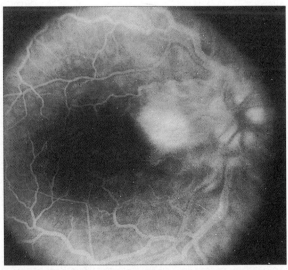

11.24 Fluorescein angiogram of patient in 11.22 six weeks later showing organization of originally noninfectious embolism, which has now formed a thickened fibrous scar on the papular–macular bundle and effectively reduced central vision to counting fingers, even though this does not result in endophthalmitis.

12.
Acquired Immune Deficiency Syndrome

Human immunodeficiency virus (HIV) is a retrovirus and has RNA as its genome. It can affect all types of human cells, but much of its pathology is secondary to infection of the T-cell helper–inducer cells. Since the T cell is crucial for the cell-mediated immune response, infection and immobilization of this cell renders a severe immunosuppression in the host. This results in opportunistic infections, which may be seen in the eye. Acquired immune deficiency syndrome (AIDS) (**Table 12.1**) is the most severe manifestation of HIV infection and occurs at a point when the immune system is rendered incompetent by the HIV infection and opportunistic organisms and infections such as *Pneumocystis carinii, Cryptococcus neoformans,* cytomegalovirus, *Toxoplasma gondii,* and candidiasis, and unusual malignancies such as Kaposi's sarcoma, may be seen (**12.1–12.8**).

The noninfectious retinopathy of AIDS may be caused by interaction between viral antigens and antibodies that circulate in the blood, but this has not been shown. The retinopathy presents as cotton wool spots without active infection and these are due to infarction of the nerve fibre layer of the retina (**12.9–12.11**). Focal microvascular dilatations may occur in the tissue adjacent to these infarctions. Usually these infarctions in the nerve fibre layer are in the order of one-quarter to one-half of a disc diameter in size and they may be distinguished from infectious retinitis by the fact that they do not enlarge and do not have cells in the vitreous overlying them. The morphology distribution of these lesions tends to change and may even disappear over a period of time. This form of retinopathy occurs in 25–90% of patients with AIDS and much less frequently in

Acquired immune deficiency syndrome (AIDS)

Definition
- Acquired immune deficiency syndrome caused by retrovirus infection (RNA only)
- Associated opportunistic infections
  Cytomegalovirus (CMV)
  Toxoplasmosis, syphilis, *Cryptococcus,* tuberculosis, *Pneumocystis*
  Other herpetic infections

Presentation
- Iridocyclitis
- Retinal cotton wool infarction early
- Retinitis late, vasculitis, necrosis

Investigation
- HIV testing
- P24 surface antigen (advanced disease)

Therapy
- Ganciclovir (CMV)
- Foscarnet (CMV)
- Peripheral retinal photocoagulation (to prevent retinal detachment)
- Acyclovir (herpetic infection)

Complications
- Retinal detachment common with CMV
- Retinal necrosis common with CMV

Prognosis
- Poor

Table 12.1 Acquired immune deficiency syndrome (AIDS).

12.1 *Pneumocystis carinii* **manifesting as choroidal tubercle** in a patient with AIDS. (Courtesy of D. Meissler, MD and C. Lowder, MD.)

patients with AIDS-related complex (ARC) or asymptomatic HIV infection.

The presence of P24 antigen, a surface HIV antigen in the blood, may also increase as the disease advances, and this may be related in time to the advancement from a cotton wool spot type of retinopathy to actual infection in the retina with an opportunistic organism. The resurgence in the general population of syphilis (**12.12–12.14**) cannot be overemphasized, particularly when occurring in conjunction with AIDS, and one should be careful to screen patients for tuberculosis as well as *Candida* and *Cryptococcus*. Both acute necrosing herpes zoster retinitis (**12.15**) and herpes simplex retinitis have

also been reported in patients with AIDS. These viral infections presenting as a necrotizing vasculitic-type retinopathy may be difficult to differentiate clinically from cytomegalovirus (CMV) retinitis. However, autopsy studies have demonstrated that more than 95% of viral retinitis in AIDS is a result of CMV infection.

In the past, patients with CMV retinitis had been immunosuppressed from cancer treatment, organ transplantation with exogenous immunosuppression from steroids and/or cyclosporin, or the immune incompetence of the newborn. CMV infection was first recognized in 1947 as a congenital infection in immunosuppressed infants. With the advent of organ

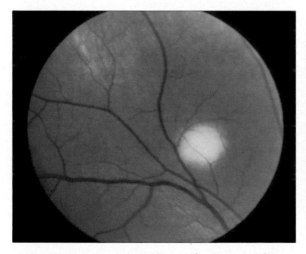

12.2 *Pneumocystis carinii* **manifesting as solitary, discrete choroidal tubercle** in a patient with AIDS. (Courtesy of D. Meissler, MD and C. Lowder, MD.)

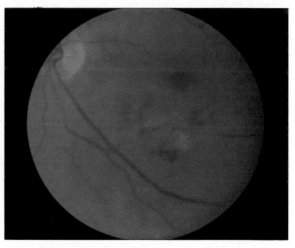

12.3 Cytomegalovirus retinitis manifesting as haemorrhagic and exudative changes.

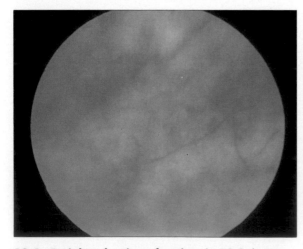

12.4 Peripheral retina of patient in 12.3 showing more extensive exudative and haemorrhagic areas of the retina.

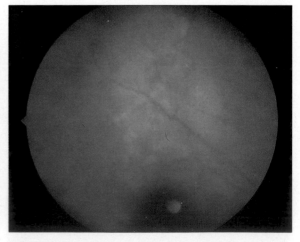

12.5 Area of retinal necrosis secondary to cytomegalovirus retinitis in a patient with AIDS.

transplantation and chemotherapy, CMV retinitis became more common in adults. It was projected that there would be 50 000 cases of CMV retinitis in 1992 as a result of AIDS alone, and this indeed proved to be the case.

Therapy of CMV retinitis used to be limited to reducing the exogenous immunosuppression of cancer and organ transplant patients. With the advent of ganciclovir (DHPG) and foscarnet, patients with AIDS could be treated. Ganciclovir is viral static, both *in vitro* and *in vivo*. Therapy with 5 mg/kg intravenously twice daily will result in more than 80% of patients having a clinical response in 10–14 days. Acyclovir is not sufficiently active against CMV infection. Recurrences are common in patients with AIDS patients due to the underlying persistent immunosuppression. Maintenance regimens are being tested for patients with AIDS, keeping them on 5 mg/kg intravenously once daily for 5–7 days/week, which may prolong the mean time for relapse. Maintenance doses lower than 25 mg/kg/week have been associated with a higher relapse rate. Foscarnet has been shown to prolong the patient's life on average four months longer than those treated with ganciclovir. Induction with 60 mg/kg/8 hours for 14 days is followed by maintenance doses of 90–120 mg/kg/day. Serum creatinine, calcium, magnesium, and haemoglobin must be followed closely for toxic effects. While the visual loss that occurred due to active infection may not improve after treatment (because of retinal necrosis), macular oedema often resolves. The main complication of ganciclovir toxicity is white cell suppression in the marrow, and white cell counts need to be checked on a weekly basis.

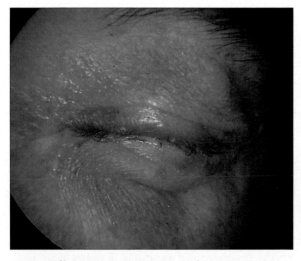

12.6   Diffuse Kaposi's sarcoma of the upper and lower eyelid of a patient with AIDS.

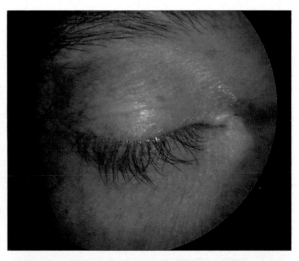

12.7   Superior palpebral infiltration by Kaposi's sarcoma.

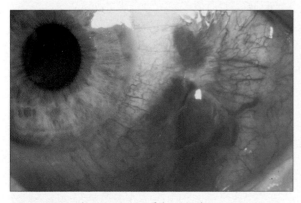

12.8   Kaposi's sarcoma of the episclera contiguous to the limbus.

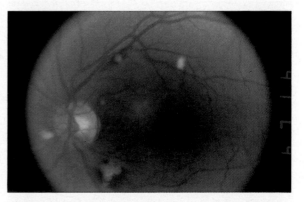

12.9   Cotton wool exudation in the nerve fibre layer of the retina indicative of infarction surrounded by minimal haemorrhage in a 28-year-old African–American male who is HIV-positive.

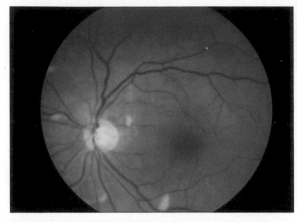

12.10   A 32-year-old white male testing HIV-positive showing multiple cotton wool exudations in the retina, but not yet having any ocular infection such as cytomegalovirus, *Pneumocystis,* or toxoplasmosis.

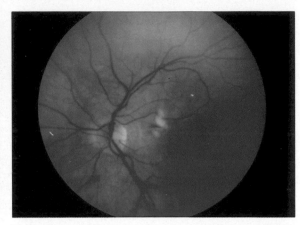

12.11   Fellow eye of patient in 12.10.

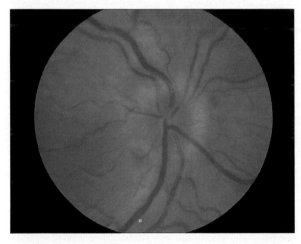

12.12   Acute papillitis in a patient who tested HIV-positive and had serology indicative of secondary syphilis infection.

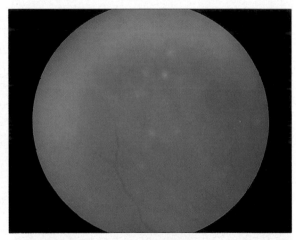

12.13   Discrete focal exudates in retina of patient who tested positive for both syphilis and HIV.

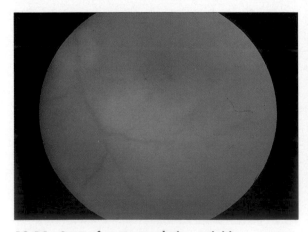

12.14   Area of acute exudative retinitis in a patient with concurrent secondary syphilis and HIV infection.

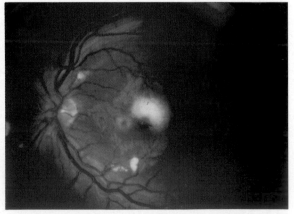

12.15   A young patient with AIDS who manifests not only cotton wool exudation in the retina, but also has acute herpes zoster retinitis. (Courtesy of Scott Wasserman, MD.)

13.
Lyme Disease

Lyme disease (**13.1–13.19, Table 13.1**) is a tick-borne spirochaetal disease caused by an organism similar to the treponeme causing syphilis. Infection with *Borrelia burgdorferi*, first identified in 1982, produces prominent symptoms and signs in the skin, heart, joints, and nervous system, as well as neuro-ophthalmological and ocular abnormalities.

Ophthalmological manifestations of Lyme disease include conjunctivitis, periocular oedema, iridocyclitis, panophthalmitis, choroiditis, optic disc swelling, macular oedema, pseudotumour cerebri, and optic neuritis, as well as optic neuropathy.

Episcleritis and conjunctivitis have been associated with each report of ocular inflammation.

It is to be noted in the literature that a positive Lyme titre, the consequence of Lyme disease, can very rarely produce a positive Venereal Disease Reference Laboratory test (VDRL), but is never responsible for a positive fluorescent treponemal antibody absorption test (FTA–ABS).

It is important to note that papilloedema is observed in association with the meningoencephalitis of Lyme disease, occasionally presenting with elevated intracranial pressure and transient visual

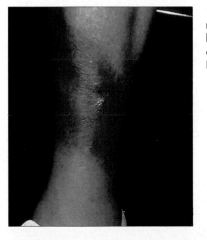

13.1 Classic round 'target' lesion on the leg of a patient with Lyme disease.

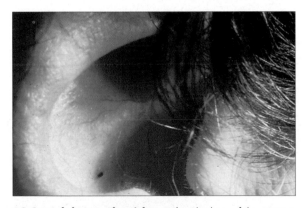

13.2 Adult *Ioxodes* tick noted in the hair of this patient with Lyme disease. (Courtesy of A.B. McDonald, MD.)

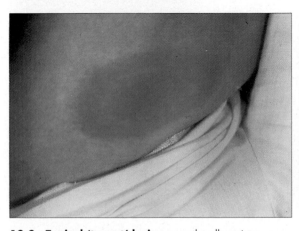

13.3 Typical 'target' lesion near the elbow in a patient with Lyme disease.

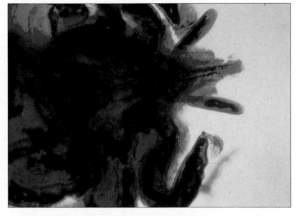

13.4 High magnification of tick in the nymphal form removed from the skin of a patient with Lyme disease.

Lyme disease

Definition
- Acute or chronic infection

Presentation
- Conjunctivitis
- Iridocyclitis
- Choroiditis
- Phthisis bulbi
- Optic nerve inflammation

Investigation
- Indirect immunofluorescent antibody (IFA)
- Enzyme-linked immunosorbent assay (ELISA) (check both IgG and IgM)
- May be negative in early disease and in cases treated early
- Medical consultation

Therapy
- Doxycycline, 100 mg twice daily
- Amoxycillin (250–500 mg twice daily)
- Penicillin G, 224 million units/day intravenously
- Ceftriaxone, 2 g/day intravenously

Complications
- Papilloedema
- Optic perineuritis
- Disc oedema
- Keratitis
- Neuritis (third and fourth nerves)

Prognosis
- Good, if treated early
- Poor, if treated late

Table 13.1   Lyme disease.

obscurations. Facial palsies, diplopia and cranial nerve deficit have repeatedly been reported with Lyme disease in the literature.

Lyme disease usually begins in the summer, less often during spring or fall, but only rarely in winter. This is due to the timing of the tick-borne infection and the tick's need for blood meals. Reported worldwide, Lyme disease has been noted in 43 American states. Most cases have clustered in a few endemic areas, mainly the Northeast, Minnesota, Wisconsin, and the West Coast.

The pathognomonic criteria for the diagnosis of Lyme disease includes the circular rash, which develops into erythema migrans following the tick bite. It enlarges, and as the centre clears, it forms an erythematous annular lesion, which is painful and itchy. The untreated lesion usually lasts several weeks, but can recur for up to a year. Unfortunately, the rash may not be seen in half the patients who present with confusing manifestations of ocular or neurological disease, which have been ascribed to Lyme disease.

The serological evidence for Lyme disease may include the enzyme-linked immunosorbent assay (ELISA) and the indirect immunofluorescent antibody (IFA). Both of these tests measure the IgM and IgG in patient's serum reacting with *B. burgdorferi*. A serum dilution greater than 1:256 is considered positive. Many patients who present with confusing ophthalmological and neurological signs may be considered to have Lyme disease. They may not be aware of a pre-existing bite of a tiny tick or having a history of

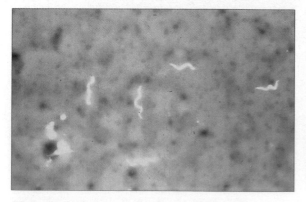

13.5   Typical spirochaete forms of *Borrelia burgdorferi*.

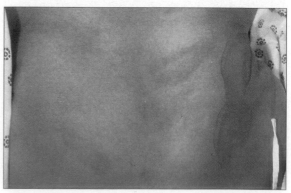

13.6   Multiple 'target' lesions on the neck of a patient with Lyme disease.

erythema migrans. The Center for Disease Control in Atlanta lists the current definition of Lyme disease including any of the following:

- A patient who lives in an endemic area with erythema migrans within 30 days of exposure to a tick bite.
- A patient exposed in an endemic area without erythema migrans, but with involvement of one organ system and a positive laboratory test.
- A patient without a history of exposure to a tick bite, but with erythema migrans as well as involvement of two organs.
- A patient without exposure in an endemic area, but with erythema migrans and positive serology.

The disease progresses through three stages.

Stage I (infection)

Stage I (infection) includes a dermatological manifestation of erythema migrans, lymphadenopathy, fever, and flu-like symptoms, which may include headache, stiff neck, and nausea. This includes the initial ophthalmological presentation of conjunctivitis, photophobia, and episcleritis.

Stage II (dissemination)

Stage II (dissemination) includes the erythema chronicum migrans, lymphocytoma, cardiac abnormalities, which include palpitations, arrhythmia, and heart block, and even mild choroiditis, as well as arthritis and arthralgias.

Disease in this stage may progress in a neurological manner to include meningitis with papilloedema, craniofacial neuritis and neuroinflammation, painful radiculopathy, and encephalitis. It is during stage II of the disease that most of the significant ophthalmological features of Lyme disease such as iritis or iridocyclitis, uveitis, retinitis, pars planitis, choroiditis, and endophthalmitis, and the neurological manifestations of optic disc swelling, optic disc pallor, optic disc inflammation, Horner's syndrome and even Argyll–Robertson pupil occur.

Stage III (late immunological disease)

Stage III or the late immunological disease includes chronic acrodermatitis atrophicans, a chronic rheumatological manifestation, with fatigue and encephalomyelitis, a demyelination syndrome suggesting multiple sclerosis, and late stromal–keratitis in the front of the eye, with episcleritis and orbital myositis.

The treatment of Lyme disease is oral tetracycline, 250 mg four times a day, or doxycycline, 100 mg twice a day for 10–30 days. For children in whom tetracycline is contraindicated, amoxycillin or penicillin G is recommended, and in cases of penicillin allergy, erythromycin proves effective.

Stage II Lyme disease may call for intravenous ceftriaxone, 2 g/day for two weeks or longer. Oral doxycycline may be substituted.

The use of corticosteroids in Lyme disease is still controversial. They have been helpful in treating choroiditis and arthritis and certain neurological sequelae, but a high incidence of failure to antibiotic treatment has been reported in patients who have been previously treated with steroids.

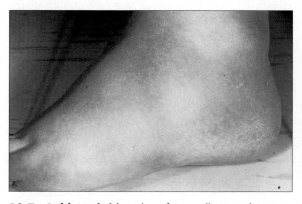

13.7 Ankle arthritis with profuse swelling, erythema and heat secondary to Lyme disease.

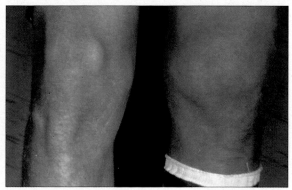

13.8 Baker's cysts and arthritis of both knees in a patient with Lyme disease.

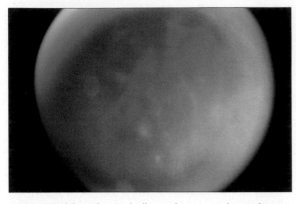

13.9 Vitritis with snowballs overlying retinal vasculitis in a patient with Lyme disease.

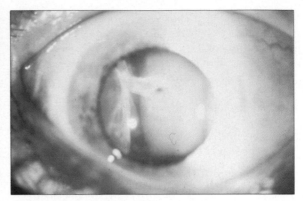

13.10 Dense vitritis behind clear lens in a patient with Lyme disease. (Courtesy of W. Culbertson, MD.)

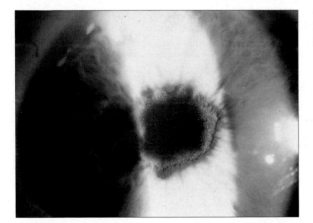

13.11 Iridocyclitis manifestations of Lyme disease with keratic precipitates and posterior synechiae. (Courtesy of W. Culbertson, MD.)

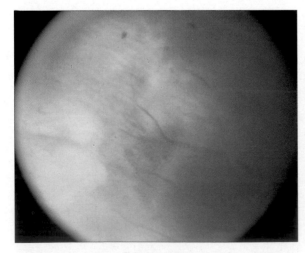

13.12 Lyme vasculitis in retina. (Courtesy of R. Nozik, MD.)

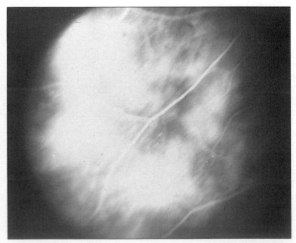

13.13 Fluorescein angiogram of patient in 13.12 highlighting the vasculitis in the retina with emphasized retinitis surrounding this, which is not as obvious in the clinical photograph.

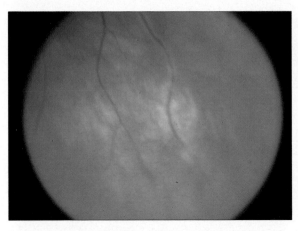

13.14   A young female patient with retinitis and vasculitis secondary to Lyme disease.

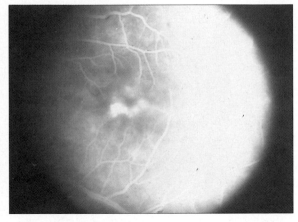

13.15   Vasculitis of the retina with retinal/choroidal inflammation highlighted on fluorescein angiogram.

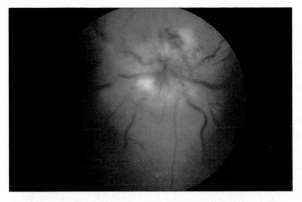

13.16   A 26-year-old white female with a haemorrhagic papillitis secondary to Lyme disease.

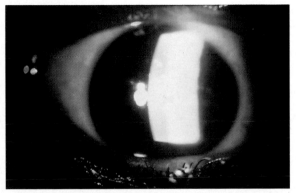

13.17   Acute iridocyclitis and corneal inflammatory changes in the stroma secondary to Lyme disease.

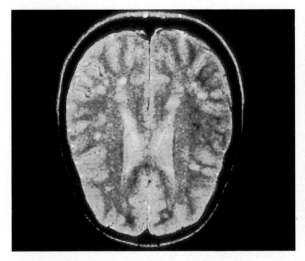

13.18   MRI of patient with small multiple inflammatory foci in the white matter of the brain secondary to Lyme encephalitis.

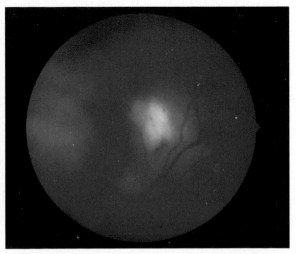

13.19   Focal area of chorioretinitis in Lyme disease.

14.
Differential Diagnosis

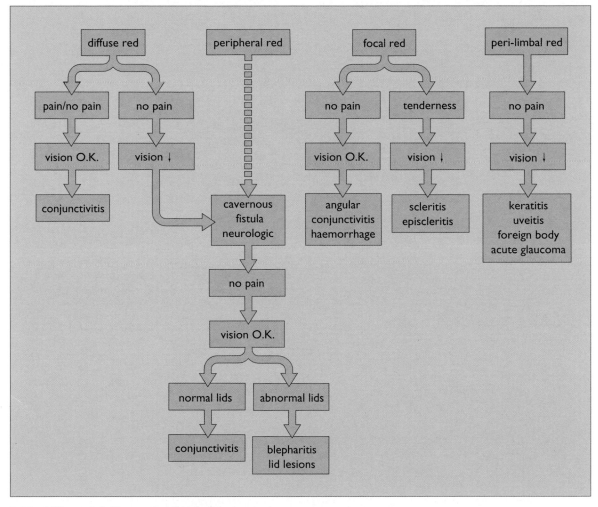

14.1 Differential diagnosis of red eye.

I. cytology findings on conjunctival scraping:				
	allergy	bacterial	viral	chlamydia
neutrophils	–	+	+	+
eosinophiles	+	–	–	+/–
lymphocytes	+	–	+	+
plasma cells	–	–	–	+
inclusions: cytoplasm	–	–	–	+
nucleus	–	–	herpetic	–

II. aetiologic considerations of discharge from eye			
discharge			
serous or "watery"	mucoid	mucopurulent	purulent
viral allergic toxic foreign body	allergic keratitis sicca	bacterial chlamydial Stevens-Johnsons syndrome	bacterial

14.2 Guidelines on the diagnosis and treatment of conjunctivitis (red eye). (Published with permission from the journal Ocular Immunology and Inflammation, Volume II, 1994, pp. 49–53, Copyright Æolus Press.)

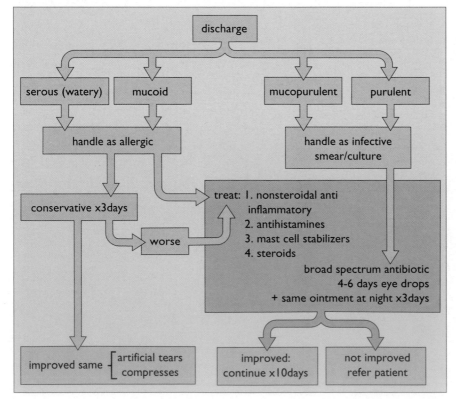

14.3 Management of conjunctivitis based upon discharge characteristics. (Published with permission from the journal Ocular Immunology and Inflammation, Volume II, 1994, pp. 49–53, Copyright Æolus Press.)

papillary	follicular	cicatricial	membranous	hemorrhagic	phlyctenules	granuloma
allergy	drug-induced	ocular cicatricial pemphigoid	microbial	viral	microbial	sarcoid
bacterial	Parinaud's syndrome	Stevens-Johnsons	toxic	irritative	immune reaction	chalazion
contact lens related	viral	irritative	Stevens-Johnsons	—	—	foreign boby
toxic	chlamydia	chemical	ligneous conjunctivitis	—	—	cat scratch disease
superior limbic conjunctivitis	—	rosacea chlamydia	ocular pemphigoid	—	—	microbial
irritative	—		chlamydia in newborn	—	—	parasitic

14.4 Conjunctival manifestations of conjunctivitis (red eye). (Published with permission from the journal Ocular Immunology and Inflammation, Volume II, 1994, pp. 49–53, Copyright Æolus Press.)

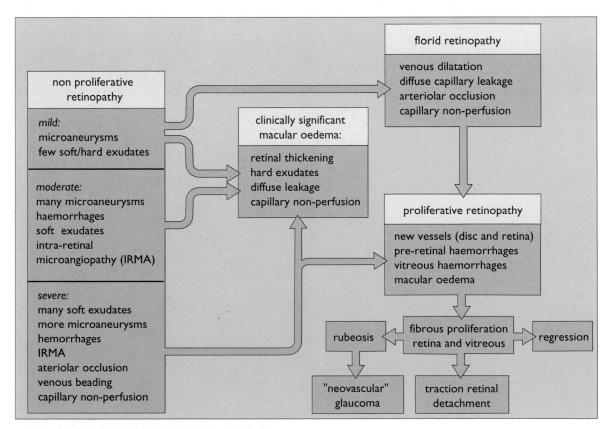

14.5 Natural history of ocular diabetic disease.

clinical status	flurescein angiography	laser treatment	other
1. normal or minimal nonproliferative retinopathy	–	–	–
2. normal or minimal nonproliferatve without macular edema	–	–	may follow with photos
3. nonproliferative retinopathy insignificant macular edema	elective	–	–
4. nonproliferatve retinopathy with macular edema	+	+ (exceptions: focal grid or pan retinal photo coag.,PRP)	–
5. severe non prolif. retinopathy	+	uncertain: focal or PRP	–
6. non-high risk prolif. diabetic retinopathy	usually	elective	occaisonal PRP
7. non-risk prolif. with macular edema	+	+	occaisonal PRP after focal Rx
8. high-risk prolif. diabetic retinopathy	usually	+	–
9. high-risk prolif. not candidate for laser	yes/no	not-possible	possible: a. pan ret cryo b. pars plana vitrectomy c. pars plana wi endolaser

14.6 Diabetic retinopathy management.

loss of vision	front of eye	middle eye	posterior eye
painful	corneal abrasion keratitis	iritis, pupillary glaucoma	pan-uveitis
	corneal ulcer	acute narrow angle glaucoma	post. scleritis
painless	conjuctivitis	secondary glaucoma	
	corneal scarring	"white eye" iridocyclitis (1,2)	vitreous (3,4,5)
		chronic open angle	retinal (6,7,8)
		glaucoma	mac. degen. choroidal (9,10)
		cateract	

14.7 Causes of loss of vision.
1: Juvenile rheumatoid arthritis
2: Large cell lymphoma
3: Haemorrhage
4: Inflammation
5: Necrosis
6: Degeneration
7: Inflammation
8: Retinal pathology
9: Macular degeneration
10: Choroidal pathology

cornea	vitreous/choroid
endothelial cell loss edema scarring band keratopathy (calcium deposition) vascularization keratic precipitates corneal decompensation	posterior vit. detachment cells in vitreous vitreous membranes atrophy/scarring choroid
anterior chamber	**retinalopic nerve**
iris scarring (1) iris neovascularization synechiae, peripheral or posterior glaucoma (2) iris necrosis/atrophy trabeculitis (3)	perivaculitis of retina macular edema retino-choroidal scarring retinal detachment retinal necrosis hyperplasia/atrophy of retinal pigment epithelium optic atrophy
lena and ciliary body	**glaucoma**
cataract hyalinization of ciliary processes proliferation of ciliary epithelium cyclitic membrane leakage of lens protein glaucoma (4)	secondary open angle or closed angle

14.8 Signs and sequlae of intraocular inflammation.

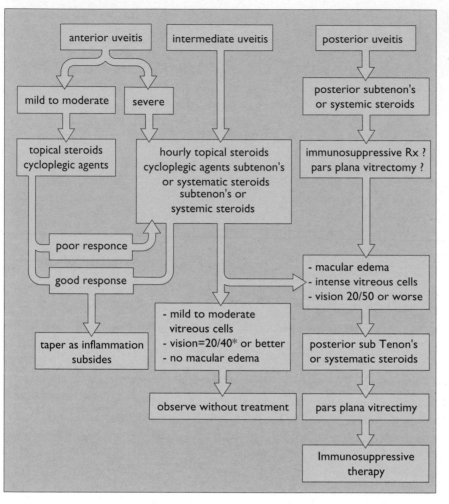

14.9 Treatment strategy for uveitis (non-specific etiology).

Selected References

TEXTBOOKS

Friedlaender MH. *Allergy and Immunology of the Eye*, 2nd Edition, Hagerstown, MD, Harper and Row, 1991.

Gold DH, Weingeist TA. *The Eye in Systemic Disease*, Philadelphia, JB Lippincott, 1990.

Michelson JB. *A Color Atlas of Uveitis*, 2nd Edition, St. Louis, Mosby, 1992.

Nussenblatt RB, Palestine AG. *Uveitis: Fundamentals and Clinical Practice*, Chicago, Yearbook Medical Publishers, Inc., 1989.

Robbins HS, Michelson JB. *Illustrated Handbook of Drug Abuse: Recognition and Diagnosis*, Chicago, Yearbook Medical Publishers, Inc., 1988.

Smith RE, Nozik RA. *Uveitis: A Clinical Approach to Diagnosis and Management*, 2nd Edition, Baltimore, Williams and Wilkins, 1991.

CHAPTER 1

Catterall RD, Perkins ES. Uveitis and urogenital disease in the male. *Br J Ophthalmol* 45: 109, 1961.

Keat A. Reiter's syndrome and reactive arthritis in perspective. *N Engl J Med* 309: 501, 1983.

Key SN, Kamura SJ. Iridocyclitis associated with juvenile arthritis. *Am J Ophthalmol* 80: 425, 1975.

Krane SM. *Rheumatoid Arthritis*, New York, Scientific American Medicine, 1985.

Scharf Y, Zonis S. Histocompatibility antigens (HLA) and uveitis. *Surv Ophthalmol* 24: 220, 1980.

Watson PG, Hayrah SS. Scleritis and episcleritis. *Br J Ophthalmol* 60: 163, 1976.

CHAPTER 2

Char DH. *Thyroid Eye Disease*, 2nd Edition, New York, Churchill-Livingstone, 1989.

Davis MD. Diabetic retinopathy: A clinical overview. Diabetes Metab Rev 4:291, 1988.

Diabetes Control and Complications Trial Research Group. Diabetes 35:530, 1986.

Diabetes Control and Complications Trial Research Group. N Engl J Med 318:246, 1988.

Diabetes Control and Complications Trial Research Group. N Engl J Med 329:977, 1993.

Duane TD. *Clinical Ophthalmology*, Volume 5, Chapters 1 and 2, Philadelphia, JP Lippincott, 1986.

Gorman CA. The presentation and management of endocrine ophthalmopathy. Clin Endocrinol Metab 7:67, 1978.

Iloaiello LM, et al. The eye and diabetes, In: Marbel A, et al. (eds), *Joslin's Diabetes Mellitus*, Philadelphia, Lea & Febiger, 1985.

Zimmerman EA. Tumors of the pituitary gland, In: Rowland LP (ed), *Merrit's Textbook of Neurology*, 7th Edition, Philadelphia, Lea and Febiger, 1984.

CHAPTER 3

Appen R, Wray S, Cogan DG. Central retinal artery occlusion. Am J Ophthalmol 79:374-381, 1975.

Arruga J, Sanders MD. Ophthalmologic findings in 70 patients with evidence of retinal embolism. Ophthalmology 88:1333-1347, 1982.

Bar CC, Green WR, Payne JW, et al. Intraocular reticulum sarcoma. Surv Ophthalmol 19:224, 1975.

Brown GC, Magargal LE, Shields JA, et al. Retinal arterial obstruction in children and young adults. Ophthalmology 88:18, 1981.

Brownstein S, et al. Atheromatous plaques of the retinal blood vessels. Arch Ophthalmol 90:49-52, 1973.

Char DH, Margolis I, Newman AB. Ocular reticulum cell sarcoma. Am J Ophthalmol 91:480, 1981.

Green WR, et al. Central retinal vein occlusion: A prospective histopathologic study of 29 eyes in 28 cases. Retina 1:27-55, 1981.

Hermans PE. The clinical manifestations of infective endocarditis. Mayo Clin Proc 57:15, 1982.

Leishman R. The eye in general vascular disease: Hypertension arteriosclerosis. Br J Ophthalmol 41:641, 1957.

Michelson JB, et al. Ocular reticulum cell sarcoma presentation as retinal detachment with demonstration of monoclonal immunoglobulin light chains on the vitreous cells. Arch Ophthalmol 99:1409, 1981.

CHAPTER 4

Chard DH, Margolis L, Newman AB. Ocular reticulum cell sarcoma. Am J Ophthalmol 91:480-483, 1981.

Chard DH, Schwartz A, Miller TR, Abele JS. Ocular metastases from systemic melanoma. Am J Ophthalmol 90:702-707, 1980.

Ferry AP, Font RL. Carcinoma metastatic to the eye orbit: A clinico-pathologic study of 227 cases. Arch Ophthalmol 92:276-286, 1974.

Ferry AP, Font RL. Carcinoma metastatic to the eye orbit: A clinico-pathologic study of 26 patients with carcinoma metastatic to the anterior segment of the eye. Arch Ophthalmol 93:472-582, 1975.

Michelson JB, Felberg NT, Shields JA. Metastatic adenocarcinoma. Am J Ophthalmol 86:142-143, 1978.

Shields JA. *Diagnosis and Management of Intraocular Tumors*, St. Louis, CV Mosby Co., 1983.

Shields JA, Michelson JB, Leonard BC, Thompson R. Retinoblastoma in an 18-year-old male. J Pediatr Ophthalmol 13:274-277, 1976.

Shields JA, Zimmerman LE. Lesions simulating malignant melanoma of the posterior uvea. Arch Ophthalmol 86:466-471, 1973.

CHAPTER 5

Cibis GW, Triphathi RC, Triphathi BJ. Glaucoma in Sturge-Weber syndrome. Ophthalmology 91:1061, 1984.

Enjolras O, Riche MC, Merland JJ. Facial port wine stains in Sturge-Weber syndrome. Pediatrics 76:48, 1985.

Font RL, Ferry AP. The phakomatoses. Int Ophthalmol Clin 12:1, 1972.

Harley RD, Baird HW, Craven EM. Ataxia-telangiectasia: Report of seven cases. Arch Ophthalmol 77:582, 1967.

Mansour AM, Wells CG, Jampole LM, et al. Ocular complications of arteriovenous communications of the retina. Arch Ophthalmol 107:232-236, 1989.

Riccardi VM. Von Recklinghausen's neurofibromatosis. N Engl J Med 305:1617-1626, 1981.

Smith JL, Cogan DG. Ataxia-telangiectasia. Arch Ophthalmol 62:364, 1959.

Williams R, Taylor D. Tuberous sclerosis. Surv Ophthalmol 30:143, 1985.

CHAPTER 6

Beutler E. Screening for galactosemia: Studies of the gene frequencies for galactosemia and the Duarte variant. Isr J Med Sci 9:1323-1329, 1973.

Beutler E, Kreill A, Cummings D, et al. Galactokinase deficiency: An important cause of familial cataracts in children and young adults. J Lab Clin Med 76:1006, 1970.

Brownstein MH, Elliott R, Helwig EB. Ophthalmologic aspects of amyloidosis. Am J Ophthalmol 69:423-430, 1970.

Burns RP. Soluble tyrosine amino transferase deficiency: An unusual case cause of corneal ulcers. Am J Ophthalmol 73:400-402, 1972.

Cogan D, Kuwabara T. The sphingolipidosis in the eye. Arch Ophthalmol 79:437-452, 1968.

Converse CA, Hammer HM, Packard CJ, et al. Plasma lipid abnormalities in retinitis pigmentosa and related conditions. Trans Ophthalmol Soc UK 103:508-512, 1983.

Fishman RS, Sunderman FW. Band keratopathy in gout. Arch Ophthalmol 75:367-369, 1966.

Kaiser-Kupfer MI, Ludweig IH, De Monasterio FM, et al. Gyrate atrophy of the choroid and retina: Early findings. Ophthalmology 92:394-401, 1985.

Lowden JA, O'Brien JS. Sialidosis: A review of human neuraminidase deficiency. Am J Hum Genet 31:1, 1979.

Macleod PM, Dolman CL, Nickel RE, et al. Prenatal diagnosis of neuronal ceroid-lipofuscinoses. Am J Med Genet 22:781, 1985.

Matot HY, et al. Frequency of carriers of chronic "type 1" Gaucher's disease in Ashkenazi Jews. Am J Med Genet 227:561-565, 1987.

Moore AT, Pritchard J, Taylor DSI. Histiocytosis X: An ophthalmologic

review. Br J Ophthalmol 69:7, 1985.

Renie WA, editor. *Goldberg's Genetic and Metabolic Eye Disease.* Boston, Little Brown and Co., 1986.

Sanderson PO, Kuwabara T, Stark W. Cystinosis: A clinical histopathologic and ultrastructural study. Arch Ophthalmol 19:272-274, 1974.

Savage DJ, Mango CA, Streeten BW. Amyloidosis of the vitreous. Arch Ophthalmol 100:1776-1779, 1982.

Sher NA, Reif FW, Watson RD, et al. Central retinal artery occlusion complicating Fabry's disease. Arch Ophthalmol 96:815-817, 1978.

Walton DS, Robb IM, Crocker AC. Ocular manifestations of group A Niemann-Pick disease. Am J Ophthalmol 85:174-180, 1978.

Wiebers DO, Hollenhorst RW, Goldstein NP. The ophthalmologic manifestations of Wilson's disease. Mayo Clin Proc 52:409-416, 1977.

Zarbin MA, Green WA, Moser H, et al. Increased levels of ceramide in the retina of a patient with Farber's disease. Arch Ophthalmol 106:1163, 1988.

CHAPTER 7

Binder PS. Herpes simplex keratitis. Surv Ophthalmol 21:313-327, 1977.

Braunstein RA, Rosan DA, Bird AE. Ocular histoplasmosis syndrome in the United Kingdom. Br J Ophthalmol 58:893, 1974.

Darell RW. Acute tuberculosis panophthalmitis. Arch Ophthalmol 78:51-54, 1967.

Dawson CR, Schachter J. Tric agent infections of the eye and genital tract. Am J Ophthalmol 63:1288, 1967.

Donahue HC. Ophthalmologic experience in a tuberculosis sanitorium. Am J Ophthalmol 64:742-748, 1967.

Ellis GH, Pakalnis VA, Worley G, et al. *Toxocara canis* infestation. Ophthalmology 93:1032, 1986.

Gass J. Ocular manifestations of acute mucor mycosis. Arch Ophthalmol 65:226, 1961.

Greenwald MJ, Wohl LG, Cell CH. Metastatic bacterial endophthalmitis: A contemporary reappraisal. Surv Ophthalmol 31:81, 1986.

Holland GN, Pepose JS, Pettit TH, et al. Acquired immune deficiency syndrome: Ocular manifestations. Ophthalmology 90:859-872, 1983.

Holland GN, Sidikero Y, Kreiger AE, et al. Treatment of cytomegalovirus retinopathy with gancyclovir. Ophthalmology 94:815-823, 1987.

Kestelyn P, Van De Pere P, Rouvroy D, et al. A prospective study of the ophthalmologic findings in the acquired immune deficiency syndrome in Africa. Am J Ophthalmol 100:230-238, 1985.

King RE, Praeger DL, Hallet JW. Amoebic choroidosis. Arch Ophthalmol 72:16-22, 1964.

Malik SRK, Gupta AK, Choudhry S. Ocular cysticercosis. Am J Ophthalmol 66:1168-1171, 1968.

Michelson JB. Infectious clinical uveitis. Curr Opin Ophthalmol 1:373-384, 1990.

Michelson JB, Belmont JB, Higgenbottom P. Juxtapupillary choroiditis associated with a chronic meningitis due to *Coccidioides immitis.* Ann Ophthalmol 15: 666-668, 1983.

Michelson JB, et al. Foreign body granuloma of the retina associated with intravenous cocaine addiction. Am J Ophthalmol 87:278, 1979.

Michelson JB, Friedlaender MH. Endophthalmitis of drug abuse. Int Ophthalmol Clin 27:120-126, 1987.

Michelson JB, Roth AM, Waring GO. Lepromatous iridocyclitis diagnosed by anterior chamber paracentesis. Am J Ophthalmol 88:674, 1979.

Michelson JB, Shields JA, McDonald PR, et al. Retinitis secondary to acquired systemic toxoplasmosis with isolation of the parasite. Am J Ophthalmol 86:548, 1978.

Oh and Jo, (eds). Symposium of herpes virus infections. Surv Ophthalmol 21:2, 1976.

Pollard ZF. ELISA for diagnosis of ocular toxocariasis. Ophthalmology 86:743, 1979.

Presley GD. Fundus changes in Rocky Mountain spotted fever. Am J Ophthalmol 67:263-264, 1969.

Saari M, et al. Acquired toxoplasma chorioretinitis. Arch Ophthalmol 94:1485, 1976.

Scholz R, Green WR, Kutys R, et al. Histoplasma capsulatum in the eye. Ophthalmology 91:1100-1104, 1984.

Taylor HR, Murphy RP, Newland HS, et al. Comparison of the treatment of ocular onchocerciasis with ivermectin and diethylcarbamazine. Arch Ophthalmol 104:863-870, 1986.

Toussaint D, Danis P. Retinopathy in generalized loa loa filariasis: A clinical pathologic study. Arch Ophthalmol 74:470-476, 1965.

Welsh HN. Bilharzial conjunctivitis. Am J Ophthalmol 66:933, 1968.

Wilhelmus KR. Ocular involvement in infectious mononucleosis. Am J Ophthalmol 89:117-118, 1981.

CHAPTER 8

Jabs DA, Johns CJ. Ocular involvement in chronic sarcoidosis. Am J Ophthalmol 102:302-107, 1986.

Masuda K. Harada's disease: A new therapeutic approach. Jpn J Clin Ophthalmol 23:553, 1969.

McLane NJ, Carroll DM. Ocular manifestations of drug abuse. Surv Ophthalmol 30:298-313, 1986.

Michelson JB, Friedlaender MH. Endophthalmitis of drug abuse. Int Ophthalmol Clin 27:120-126, 1987.

Michelson JB, Freedman SD, et al. Aspergillus endophthalmitis in a drug abuser. Ann Ophthalmol 14:1051-1054, 1982.

Michelson JB, Robin HS. *Illustrated Handbook of Drug Abuse: Recognition and Diagnosis*, Chicago, Yearbook Medical Publishers, Inc., 1988.

Michelson JB, Robin HS, Nozik RE. Nonocular manifestations of parenteral drug abuse (Reviews in medicine). Surv Ophthalmol 30:314, 1986.

Michelson JB, Whitchard P, et al. Possible foreign body granuloma of the retina associated with intravenous cocaine addiction. Am J Ophthalmol 87:278-280, 1979.

Obenauf CD, Shaw HE, Sydnor CF, Klintworth GK. Sarcoidosis and its ophthalmic manifestations. Am J Ophthalmol 86:684-695, 1978.

O'Duffy, Kokmane. *Behçet's Disease: Basic and Clinical Aspects*, New York, Marcel Dekker, Inc., 1991.

Ohno S, Kimura SJ, O'Connor GR. Vogt-Koyanagi-Harada syndrome. Am J Ophthalmol 83:735, 1977.

Rosen VJ. Cutaneous manifestations of drug abuse by parenteral injections. Am J Dermatopathol 7:79-83, 1985.

CHAPTER 9

Michelson JB. Melting cornea with collapsing nose (relapsing polycondritis): A clinical pathologic relation. Surv Ophthalmol 29:148, 1984.

Michelson JB, Chisari FV. Behçet's disease: A review. Surv Ophthalmol 26:190, 1982.

CHAPTER 10

Fraunfelder FT, Roy H, (eds). Dermatologic disorders, In: *Current Ocular Therapy*, 4th Edition, Philadelphia, WB Saunders, pp. 200-224, 1995.

Friedlaender MH. Disorders of the eye, In: Orkin M, Maibach HI, Dahl MV (eds), *Dermatology*, Norwalk, Appleton & Lange, 1991.

Friedlaender MH. *Allergy and Immunology of the Eye*, 2nd Edition, New York, Raven, pp. 75-106, 1993.

Leisegang TJ, (ed). Oculodermal Diseases, Ophthalmol Clin N Am, 1992.

Ostler HB. *Diseases of the External Eye and Adnexa*, Baltimore, Williams & Wilkins, pp. 712-738, 1993.

CHAPTER 11

Friedlaender MH. Contact allergy and toxicity in the eye. Int Ophthalmol Clin 28:317-320, 1989.

Ostler HB. *Diseases of the External Eye and Adnexa*, Baltimore, Williams & Wilkins, pp. 101-126, 1993.

Roberson MC. Irritative conjunctivitis, In: Fraunfelder FT, Roy H (eds), *Current Ocular Therapy*, 4th Edition, Philadelphia, WB Saunders, pp. 469-470, 1995.

Smolin G, O'Connor GR. *Ocular Immunology*, 2nd Edition, Boston, Little Brown and Co., pp. 238-242, 1986.

CHAPTER 12

Holland GN, Pepose JS, Pettit TH. Acquired immune deficiency syndrome: Ocular Manifestations. Ophthalmology 90:859-872, 1983.

Holland GN, Sitticaro Y, Kreiger AE, et al. Treatment of cytomegalovirus retinopathy with gancyclovir. Ophthalmology 94:815-823, 1987.

Palastine AG, Rodrigues MM, Macher AM, et al. Ophthalmic involvement in acquired immune deficiency syndrome. Ophthalmology 91:1092-1099, 1984.

Pepose JS, Holland GN, Nestor MS, et al. Acquired immune deficiency syndrome: Pathogenic mechanisms of ocular disease. Ophthalmology 92:472-484, 1985.

CHAPTER 13

Bertuch AW, Rocco EE, Schwartz EG. Eye findings in Lyme disease. Conn Med 51: 151, 1987.

Meyerhoff J. Lyme disease. Am J Med 75:663, 1983.

Schechter SL. Lyme disease associated with optic neuropathy. Am J Med 81:143, 1986.

Wu G, Lincoff H, Elsworth RM, et al. Optic disk edema in Lyme disease. Ann Ophthalmol 18:252, 1986.

Index